Fostering Learning in Small Groups

A Practical Guide

Jane Westberg

Hilliard Jason

Springer Publishing Company, Inc.
536 Broadway
New York, N.Y. 10012-3955

Cover design by Tom Yabut
Production Editor: Pamela Lankas

00 01 02 / 6 5 4

Library of Congress Cataloging-in-Publication Data

Westberg, Jane.
      Fostering learning in small groups : a practical guide / Jane Westberg,
   Hilliard Jason.
            p.   cm.— (Springer series on medical education)
      Includes bibliographical references and index.
      ISBN 0-8261-9331-5
         1. Medicine—Study and teaching.   2. Group work in education.
   I. Jason, Hilliard, 1933– . II. Title.   III. Series.
   R834.W475, 1996   96–1996
   610′ . 71′ 1—dc20   CIP

Printed in the United States of America

This book is gratefully dedicated to the many highly devoted teachers in the health professions who, despite minimal rewards or support from their institutions for doing so, give generously and continuously to the fortunate learners with whom they work.

Contents

List of Appendixes

Foreword

How do students learn? One would think with centuries of education behind us, the answer would be apparent to instructors everywhere. In fact, a great deal is known about the learning and teaching processes, but health professional education, for the most part, employs techniques that do not reflect that knowledge. Large group lectures are still used to "impart" detailed facts. Health professional educators, for the most part, do not make use of multiple methods of instruction designed to match individual student learning needs. Also ignored is the fact that active learning has proved to be more efficacious than passive methods. The reasons for these discrepancies are outlined in this text, but bear emphasis here.

Most health professional educators have not been educated in pedagogy. Many, if not most, were selected on the basis of criteria other than preparation for, or demonstrated excellence in, teaching modalities that reflect the best methods for learning. Research accomplishment, clinical skill, or other attributes counted more than did teaching ability or potential. Economy of instructor time also inhibits employment of effective educational methods: it is "easier" for a single faculty member to "instruct" a large group of students than for multiple instructors to teach many small groups or for a single teacher to take the time to prepare other types of educational materials, for example, interactive computerized programs, multimedia presentation, and, so on. Despite these claims that argue for continuation of less effective teaching/learning encounters, there are persuasive reasons for health professionals to use the more efficacious means for learning.

If the object of instruction is truly learning, rather than instructor convenience, then well-planned small group instruction is worth the extra effort. Westberg and Jason demonstrate ways to make small group instruction efficient in order for the students to obtain the benefits of learning in the first place. Further, the small group method allows for a variety of different types of instruction, which enhances the goals of education.

A major reason for the publication of this text is to provide knowledgeable advice, expert guidance, and reasoned approaches to the methods that the authors advocate. Both authors are experienced educators who have often been at the forefront of instructional methodology. Their experience places them in an excellent position to provide, in this text, the basic ingredients for the novice health professional instructor and ready reference for those who have some experience but wish to hone their skills. The accomplished instructor in small group settings will find this book a compendium of useful actions, not all of which one might have known or employed in the past.

Westberg and Jason provide a most complete guide to small group content, indicating how it can be used for communication skills, for problem solving, for enhancing clinical judgment, for honing attitudes, and for a variety of other desired educational outcomes. The text is replete with practical, down-to-earth information that even discusses the appropriate physical space and arrangement that facilitiates the purpose of the small group.

The sections on preparing oneself for small group sessions takes the instructor through the mind-set, the mechanics, the techniques one can employ, and the desired goals. Along the way, one learns how to monitor progress, provide feedback, and facilitate the students' achievement of the desired goals. The authors provide advice as to the commonest pitfalls: what they are and what you can do about preventing or remediating them.

I find this text a most valuable contribution to the educational literature for health professionals. One might parallel the advertising slogan by saying, "Don't begin instruction without it!"

VINCENT A. FULGINITI, MD
Chancellor and Professor of Pediatrics
University of Colorado Health Sciences Center

Introduction

For many compelling reasons, growing numbers of schools in the health professions are increasing the proportion of learning time their students spend in small groups. This book responds to that trend and is intended for a variety of educators who have interests in education in the small group setting—those who are newly serving as small group leaders; those experienced small group teachers who want to review their current approaches and enhance their skills; and those whose responsibilitites include helping others become effective small group leaders. In addition, those educators who want to persuade administrators and others of the potential value of small group teaching will find multiple arguments in support of this instructional strategy. Although we focus on educating health professionals, the principles and many of the approaches presented apply equally to educating other professionals.

THE AREAS OF FOCUS

Part I of this book (Chapters 1–5), deals with generic concepts and issues, focusing primarily on the rationale for and practical strategies involved in planning and facilitating learning in small groups. Part II (Chapters 6–10) is devoted to the process of planning for and leading small groups devoted to specific purposes, such as providing a forum for discussion and dialogue, helping learners develop interpersonal skills, or helping learners reflect on patient care experiences.

Reasons for fostering learning in small groups

During our several decades of conducting faculty development workshops and seminars for educators in the health professions we've heard many questions and concerns about the justification for and process of small group teaching. Some educators aren't convinced that small groups are useful, saying things like, "In small groups, students just share their ignorance." Or, "Lectures are more efficient than small groups. They require fewer teachers." Others want to do small group teaching but can't convince their administrators to support this approach. We respond to such concerns in several places. In Chapter 1 we present a generic rationale for small group education, discuss the characteristics of effective groups, and emphasize the importance of using a collaborative approach. In Chapters 6–10 we provide some additional, specific arguments in support of five particular ways in which small groups can be used.

Preventing and dealing with problems

During our faculty development workshops and consultations, we've often heard such misgivings as, "What if I can't get students to talk?" "How do I get a session started?" "What if some learners try to dominate the session?" "What if students get into conflicts with each other?" "What if some students don't do their fair share?" In this book we deal with such concerns and questions. We also respond to concerns that grow out of our many observations of teachers at work (e.g., Jason, 1962, 1964; Jason & Westberg, 1982).

Largely, our approach is to try helping readers prevent problems from occurring in the first place. We have found that when educators attend to needed preparatory tasks and take time to reflect in advance on the leadership tasks they will face, they have fewer problems and feel more able to deal with whatever challenges arise. In Chapter 2 we discuss such preparatory tasks as determining or clarifying who the learners are, what their learning needs are likely to be, what their roles and responsibilities will be, and if and how the learners will be evaluated. In Chapter 3 we discuss how leaders can also benefit by reflecting on what they personally can bring to groups and the kind of leadership they want to provide.

Small group sessions that include the active participation of learners are complex human events. They can be full of surprises and seem disorganized, even chaotic, at times. Much of the resulting "messiness" turns out to be necessary and desirable. Even with a skillful leader, small groups seldom proceed neatly from one topic to another in scripted lecture style. In fact, they shouldn't. As we discuss, the authoritarian, controlling leadership strategies that keep groups from experiencing any turmoil can also keep them from the meaningful, lasting learning we assume you are seeking. In Chapter 4, we try to bring some order to the seeming chaos by describing tasks and strategies that can provide a systematic way of thinking about groups and group leadership. These tasks include building trusting relationships, fostering collaboration, assessing learners' needs, clarifying or developing learning goals, deciding how to work together, facilitating the learners' active participation, monitoring and facilitating the flow of the sessions, managing conflict, and "processing" and summarizing what occurred during the session.

Under many circumstances, coleadership of small groups can offer advantages, including opportunities for interdisciplinary teaching and learning. In Chapter 5, we discuss the rationale for coleadership and suggest some tasks that can help make the experience successful.

As mentioned, Chapters 6–10 focus on five distinct small group purposes. In practice, some groups focus on only one of these purposes whereas others have several purposes. Chapters 6–10 build on the first part of the book and are not intended to be read alone. In each chapter we suggest some specific strategies for accomplishing the generic tasks outlined in Chapters 2 through 4. We also discuss some additional tasks that pertain to the purpose in question. Because tasks, such as building trust, fostering collaboration, orienting learners, and providing feedback need to be discussed in relation to all the group purposes addressed in Chapters 6–10, there is some inescapable redundancy. To minimize unnecessary repetition and keep the book from growing too large, we don't expand on issues each time we introduce them. Whenever appropriate, we refer readers to fuller explanations in earlier chapters and to the fairly detailed index.

Making decisions

The process of small group leadership, like the process of patient care, involves recognizing and responding appropriately to multiple, sequential decision points. Experience and skill are needed for recognizing decision points when they emerge. When events (branch points) requiring choices are missed, decisions still get made; but they are made inadvertently or by default, rather than by careful thought or reflection. Such decisions rarely include the best of the available options. Two major goals of this book are to help readers (a) be aware of the many decisions that are needed in preparing for and facilitating small groups and (b) have a basis for making appropriate selections among the available choices.

Please note that the suggestions we make in this book are not cookbook-type recipes for effective group leadership. Effective teaching and learning can't be reduced to precise steps and exact ingredients. Rather—continuing with the cooking metaphor—we recommend some ingredients to consider. Each instructional group session, however, is unique. Creative teaching, like creative cooking, requires improvisation and artistry, sometimes even inventing elements of the process as you go along.

LANGUAGE AND ILLUSTRATIONS USED IN THIS BOOK

This book is intended for educators in all the health professions. We have tried being as generic as possible, and we've sought to have a sufficient range of examples to provide most readers with at least some familiar events that relate to situations in which they teach. Even if some illustrations are not particularly germane to your instructional tasks, we hope you will agree that the principles behind the illustrations are fully applicable to all the health professions and beyond.

In an attempt to speak to a range of educators, we use inclusive, generic terms, a few of which we have redefined. *Learners* imply undergraduate students, graduate students, postgraduate students (including residents and house officers), fellows, and in some cases, practicing professionals who are participating in continuing education programs. The terms *health professionals*, *practitioners*, and *clinicians* are used interchangeably and include all professionals who provide health and medical care, including mental health care.

Most often we refer to people who are seeking and receiving health care as patients, but the term *clients* could be substituted. Some people consider the term *patient* to be associated with an authoritarian form of care in which people are treated as passive recipients of care rather than as partners in their care. As you will see, we strongly advocate a collaborative model in both health care and education.

We have not found an adequate, compact substitute for the word *case*. We recognize that this word is sometimes used by others in impersonal, dehumanizing ways. When we use the word, please understand that we are referring respectfully to the patient/client involved. Whenever possible, we avoid gender specificity and such awkward constructions as *herself/himself* and *his/hers*, by using plurals. Otherwise we try to alternate the use of male and female pronouns.

Finally, we know that different people have different associations with the various labels used for those who are responsible for small groups. Some people resist the word *leader*, because it connotes for them an authoritarian, even dictatorial, style that they reject. For them, the label *facilitator* may be closer to the collaborative style they prefer, while for others this latter label connotes a nondirective, even wishy-washy, style that they find unappealing. We ask you to try suspending your current associations with these and other labels and focus instead on the actual strategies that you can use to achieve a variety of purposes. We use several labels interchangeably throughout the book, meaning to imply that none is necessarily or exclusively associated with any particular instructional style.

A NOTE TO OUR READERS

We are aware that there is a wide range of experience, perspectives, and backgrounds among those who are potential readers of this book. Highly experienced teachers may find some of the material redundant. Yet, we hope that beginners find some of this purposeful repetition reinforcing and clarifying. If you are a seasoned teacher, we ask that you bear with us and use the many headers and subheaders we've included to help you navigate to those sections that are of most interest to you.

You may also conclude that some of the steps and strategies we recommend are simply reasonable and obvious. We urge you to resist any conclusion that their being logical makes them easy to implement. Even if some seem logical and self-evident, we urge you to ask yourself whether you truly do these things in your daily teaching. If you don't, we emphasize, as we will again from time to time in the text, that making changes in your ways of teaching will likely take far more than merely reading about some ideas in a book. In our work with thousands of teachers we have been consistently struck that hours of repeated practice can be needed before new approaches begin to become part of their available repertoire. In the thick of daily work, most of us revert to deeply ingrained habits. We simply don't mobilize new approaches that we've recently been exposed to but have not yet self-consciously practiced. Even after considerable practice you may find, as we do, that considerable vigilance can be needed to avoid back-sliding.

So, please find ways to think repeatedly about, discuss with colleagues, and practice often any approaches you find compelling. They are not likely to stay with you without these extra efforts, no matter how reasonable they may seem during a quick reading.

LITERATURE ON SMALL GROUPS AND OTHER MODELS

Aside from the published research of the last decade in problem-based, small group learning, relatively little has been written about the use of small groups in health professions education. We do refer to this literature but also refer to literature from a variety of other fields (e.g., organizational development, educational psychology).

Although many of the tasks and strategies that we discuss can be adapted to large groups, our primary focus here is on groups of roughly 15 students or less. Yet, some teachers are faced with groups of 25 students or more. Some even seek to bring interactive approaches to quite large groups (over 100). We discuss strategies for making interactive presentations to large groups elsewhere (Westberg & Jason, 1991a). For teachers of large groups who want to use the case-based discussion method, we recommend a helpful book by Christensen and colleagues (1991).

Some teachers break their large groups into several small groups that are led by more advanced students, or the students in the groups provide their own leadership. The tasks and strategies in this book are relevant for anyone who is serving as a leader. Indeed, one of the themes of this book is the importance of giving students increasing responsibility for the leadership of their groups. However, readers who are particularly interested in student-run groups might turn to the rather extensive literature on cooperative learning, especially more recent resources that apply to higher education (e.g., Johnson, Johnson, & Smith, 1991). (Most of the cooperative learning literature focuses on elementary and secondary education.)

Acknowledgments

This book is about the benefits and strategies of using small groups for helping others learn. Most of our attempts to teach about these and related matters have been in small group settings. At the risk of appearing to be mouthing an overworked cliché, we must explain that much of what appears in this book we learned from that work with those who were our "students." In several places in this book we've asserted that a major benefit of teaching in small groups is the learning opportunities such efforts present to the educator. We feel that we are living examples of the truth of that assertion. The many educators in the health professions with whom we have been privileged to work over the course of several decades have been an endless source of ideas, questions, surprises, challenges, and inspiration. They have provoked us to think about and study the processes we seek to convey in this document. We wish we could personally convey to all those faculty members with whom we've worked how very grateful we are for their inquisitiveness, energy, and imagination. We can only hope that they learned as much from those experiences as we did. Here we've tried to distill the essence of what those learners taught us, together with what we've derived from the many authors we cite, and from multiple others with whom we've worked, who we've not had space to cite, but whose presence is evident throughout.

We are especially grateful for the guidance we've received in refining this manuscript from our generous and perceptive reviewers. They were DeWitt C. Baldwin, Jr., MD; Howard Barrows, MD; Lucy Candib, MD; Barbara Carpio, RN; Francine Hekelman, PhD, RN; Jacob Jacobson, MD; Jill McNamara, MA; Ann O'Brien, RN, MSN; Joan Onder, MSW; Mary Ann Shea, PhD; LuAnn Wilkerson, EdD; and Patricia Williams, MD.

In this our third opportunity to work with the people of Springer Publishing Company, we extend a special thanks to those with whom we have collaborated most closely: Steven Jonas, MD, Series Editor for the Medical Education Series; Bill Tucker, Senior Editor; Ruth Chasek, Nursing Editor; Barbara Barnum, RN, PhD, FAAN; Bob Kowkabany and

Louise Farkas, Production Managers, and Pam Lankas, Production Editor. Their professionalism and dedication to helping enhance educational programs in the health professions has made this effort, yet again, a pleasure. We add a special thanks to Ursula Springer, PhD, our publisher, for the commitment, perseverance, and risk-taking she has demonstrated in providing this important and unique venue for educational books in the health professions.

JANE WESTBERG PhD and HILLIARD JASON, MD, EdD
Boulder, Colorado

1

Generic Concepts and Issues

CHAPTER 1

Small Groups in Health Professions Education

As educators in the health professions we are charged with preparing health professionals who will be competent throughout their careers—not a minor challenge in the rapidly changing world of health care. Our graduates must have a variety of well-developed capabilities (intellectual, interpersonal, manual, sensory), a considerable body of information and understandings, the ability to work collaboratively with colleagues and patients, and the skills for teaching colleagues, patients, families, and others. In addition, to remain competent for a lifetime, they need effective learning skills, an openness to learning from colleagues and patients, and a capacity to change (Westberg & Jason, 1993).

How can we best prepare our learners to be competent health professionals? Until recently a primary strategy in many health professions schools and graduate programs was the traditional lecture (a monologue that sometimes concludes with a brief period for questions from learners and answers from the teacher).[1] Learners spent large portions of their professional education (especially in the early years of their professional education) passively listening to lectures in classrooms and conference rooms. Even during small groups and clinical supervision, they were often given minilectures. These approaches, of course, are still substantial components of many courses and programs.

Researchers have documented what many educators have known intuitively: although traditional lectures can serve some useful purposes un-

---

[1] We use the phrase *traditional lecture* to identify events that contrast with highly interactive large group presentations that are usually also referred to as lectures.

der some circumstances (Westberg & Jason, 1991a), they don't provide many of the conditions or opportunities needed for fostering meaningful, lasting learning. For learning to survive and be of later use, it needs to be acquired in a context that links to the real-world situation in which it will later be put to use. Learners need to care about—have a sense of ownership of—the learning goals and strategies and even participate in developing them. They need many opportunities to practice the capabilities they are to acquire, to use their new knowledge in multiple circumstances, to reflect on and critique their experiences and practice, to invite and integrate feedback from others, to review their progress, to develop new learning goals for themselves, and more. Also, if learners are to work and learn together as practitioners, they need to practice working and learning together during their basic professional education. If students are to become active lifelong learners, they need to develop and practice the skills of effective, self-initiated learning. In short, we can't package learning and give it to learners. We can—indeed, we are obliged to—guide and facilitate our students in doing their own learning, and we need to create the conditions and opportunities that foster this learning. However, learners must be active participants in shaping and directing their learning and in building and integrating new knowledge and capabilities.

How do we provide these conditions and opportunities? Clearly, there is no single way. Different learning goals require different strategies, and students learn in a range of ways, so using a variety of learning formats is desirable. In general, as national panels of health professions educators have recommended,[2] we need to increase opportunities for students to be active learners and reduce the amount of time they are expected to listen passively to others. If we choose or are assigned to work with large groups of students, we need to make these sessions as interactive as possible. And in many institutions we need to increase the time that learners spend in supervised clinical practice, small groups, and independent study.

In this book, we focus on collaborative, interactive small groups, a learning format that is gradually becoming more widespread in health professions education. We propose that such small groups should be a central modality in all our educational programs. In this chapter we introduce reasons why these kinds of groups, of which there are several subforms, enable us to provide many of the conditions and opportunities that students need for lasting learning, especially of some vital capabilities, such as

---

[2] See, for example, The panel on the general professional education of the physician and college preparation for medicine, 1984.

being effective learners, working and learning effectively with others, and performing a variety of clinical skills.

Deciding to teach in small groups is the first step in the never-ending process of becoming a progressively better small group leader. Effective small group leaders have many capabilities: an understanding of the psychology of learning, of group processes, and of the tasks that need to be accomplished; the ability to help create an interactive, collaborative community of learners; and the capacity to "process" information rapidly and to recognize and respond to the variety of challenges that arise, making on-the-spot decisions, selecting among and inventing optional strategies. Being a small group facilitator is part science, part art. It can be exciting and rewarding to those who are prepared. For those who are not prepared, the many challenges can be unpleasantly overwhelming. When insufficiently prepared or adept, some teachers convert their small groups to something far less effective, often some variation on teacher-dominated traditional lectures or unfocused group musings.

Throughout this book we suggest ways to be well prepared for, and to derive joy from, leading small groups. In the balance of this chapter, we discuss

- reasons for using small groups to foster learning
- the importance of using a collaborative approach
- additional characteristics of effective small groups.

REASONS FOR USING SMALL GROUPS TO FOSTER LEARNING

Here we present general reasons for using small groups in educating health professionals. These arguments are likely to be of particular interest to readers who are responsible for planning instruction and want to review what can be accomplished in small groups, readers who are new to and are preparing for small group teaching, and readers who want to persuade colleagues or learners of the value of small groups. Since in many courses and schools debates continue as to whether to use traditional lectures or small groups, and whether the resource demands of small groups are justified, we occasionally contrast the two methods. We present four categories of reasons for teaching in small groups:

1. what learners need for meaningful, lasting learning
2. the benefits of peer learning

3. ways that the group setting can enable us to be more effective teachers

4. positive spin-offs that can derive from group learning.

Here we discuss what potentially can occur in small groups when planned and implemented effectively, not what necessarily or automatically happens whenever a leader and a small group of learners meet.

In small groups we can provide learners with what they need for meaningful, lasting learning

To become and remain competent health professionals, learners need the specific conditions and opportunities that are associated with meaningful, lasting learning.[3] As follows, we briefly describe the conditions and opportunities that can be provided in small groups, give reasons for why each is important, and then indicate how small groups are well suited for providing these conditions/opportunities. We expand on all of these issues later in the book.

Learners can gain a sense of "ownership" of their learning.   Students are unlikely to pursue learning goals that they feel are inconsistent with their own long-term purposes. The short-term goal of passing exams, in the absence of longer-term justifications, tends not to produce lasting learning. Learners are also unlikely to engage fully in learning strategies that they don't think are related to their needs. Learners are most likely to feel a sense of ownership of those learning goals and strategies that they have helped identify and which they feel are linked to their real learning needs.[4]

When preparing to give traditional lectures, teachers typically decide independently what they will teach, with little or no information about

---

[3] For various perspectives on these conditions and opportunities, see Knowles, 1978; Kolb, 1984; and Westberg & Jason, 1993.

[4] If you are unconvinced of the validity of these observations, think of some of the early courses in your own professional education. Did any of them feel like part of an obstacle course or a rite of passage, rather than a genuine part of your career development? If any did, they probably illustrate the point. Either those courses were truly not relevant to your career or your teachers failed in their basic instructional responsibility of helping you gain a sense of ownership of what they proposed to offer. In some programs so many courses feel irrelevant that many learners and teachers come to assume that such is the inherent nature of education, especially during the early years of professional preparation. Bad education, conducted consistently for a sufficient number of years can take on the aura of worthy tradition. We invite you to suspend any such assumptions you may have. As demonstrated by a growing number of schools, education at all levels can be genuinely relevant and exciting.

their learners' actual needs. The instructional strategies they use are selected more on the basis of habit or tradition than careful consideration of their learners' characteristics or documented needs. Not surprisingly, in such situations not all learners feel ownership of the goals or the process. In contrast, small group learning, properly conducted, depends on the active involvement of the participants in content selection and strategy design. Groups don't work unless members are committed to the session's learning goals and strategies. (In Chapter 4, we discuss ways to involve learners in planning group sessions.)

Learners can build and "metabolize" knowledge. John Dewey (1938) and Jerome Bruner (1966), like many others, have emphasized the importance of learners making their own discoveries and doing their own inquiries. As Christensen says (1991), students need "to discover for themselves rather than accept verbal or written pronouncements. They must explore the intellectual terrain without maps, step by step, blazing trails, struggling past obstacles, dealing with disappointments" (pp. 16–17). We can't give learners lasting knowledge; they must build it themselves.[5] They can memorize information that we or others have conveyed, and retain it long enough to pass conventional examinations, but, as so many clinical teachers have discovered, learners often can't recall and use this information reliably when later faced with real-life problems. To help ensure that this knowledge is retained and available when needed, learners need to learn it in a context that is as close as possible to the real-world experiences they are having or will have (Jason, 1970; Brown, Collins, & Duguid, 1989); link it to what they already know; "elaborate" on it—connect it with other knowledge areas; and use it in multiple ways on many occasions, creating a web (a structure) of deep, rich connections.[6]

In contrast to what learners need, traditional lectures often foster passivity and dependency. They typically provide answers rather than questions and create the impression that knowledge can be successfully dumped into learners' heads, like water into a bucket.[7] During uninterrupted

---

[5] See Whitman (1993) for an overview of "cognitive constructivism," an educational theory that maintains that individuals must develop their own models of reality using both personal experience and external data. For a fuller discussion of this theory and its implications, see Fosnot (1989).

[6] For more on the concept of elaboration, see Coles (1991), and Norman and Schmidt (1992), and the references they cite.

[7] The inappropriateness of the pace and the process of these efforts at knowledge transfer was colorfully captured by David Rogers (while President of the Robert Wood Johnson Foundation) in his observation that learning in many courses is like having to drink from a fire hose (1982).

lectures, learners are discouraged or prevented from reflecting on or challenging ideas, even internally. If they become reflective during a lecture, they are likely to suffer by missing the teacher's next points. Even when the lecture sessions include opportunities for questions, the time for such interactions is typically brief and dominated by a subset of learners (Karp & Yoels, 1987). Much of the meaningful learning that occurs in courses taught by traditional lecturing appears to derive from the studying learners do afterward, alone, and with others. The central benefit offered by many lectures is the transmission of the teacher's expectations, which then guide the students' studies, a task that could be accomplished at least as well and less ambiguously with a written handout, saving everyone a good deal of time.[8]

In the kinds of small groups we emphasize in this book, learning takes place within a context that evokes and encourages the learners' questions. The context might be a case created by the teacher, an experience learners engage in during the group (e.g., a role play), or one of the learner's actual patient care experiences. As learners reflect on and discuss these events, they typically dig into their own experiences and understandings, offer what they think might be relevant, examine their own and each other's ideas and assumptions, elaborate on what they are learning, and identify what they still need to learn. Particularly if the group is meeting only once, additional information might be available to learners during the group session. (Books, journals, and computers might be in the room. In some cases, the teacher might serve as a resource.) When the group will be meeting multiple times, the learners might be responsible for gathering information outside of the group (from the library and/or consultants) and bringing this information back to the next session to use in the group's continuing reflections, problem solving, or other tasks. In other words, learners engage in the steps needed for genuine learning. [9,10]

Learners can observe and practice needed capabilities. For

---

[8]Since teachers often derive benefits from the lectures they attend, many conclude that lectures are valuable; more so than they often turn out to be for their students. As experts in their fields, teachers bring to the lectures they attend a considerable "readiness" for what is presented (questions in their heads that are answered by the lecturer). Most of their students, being relative beginners, don't bring this readiness to the lectures they attend. Further, the lectures attended by teachers typically convey general concepts, recent findings, or intriguing history, not abundant detail on which they will later be tested.

[9] These steps closely parallel those of the "adult learning cycle," proposed by Kolb (1984).

[10] Many students intuitively recognize that these steps are needed for learning and try to add them to their experiences in lecture-based courses. If time is available, and the program hasn't caused too much of a sense of competition among the learners, they form their own after-hours small groups in which they test their understandings and try to link new material to what they already know.

learners to acquire and retain capabilities, they need to practice doing them, repeatedly and systematically, and, at least initially, under supervision. But first, learners need clear images of the capabilities they are to develop. Generally they form these images by observing their teachers or others modeling or demonstrating these skills, preferably while providing explanations. Complex capabilities are usually learned most effectively in stages. An optimal approach provides practice initially in a safe, simulated setting; then practice in a real clinical situation under supervision, with relatively uncomplicated versions of the task, or with manageable pieces of the task; then further practice for refinement in a simulated setting; then practice again under supervision in a clinical setting with a higher level challenge, and so on (Westberg & Jason, 1993). This staged learning can be further helped by alternating this practice with demonstrations provided in response to the learners' requests. These interplays of observation and practice are especially important when students are learning a complex performing art, as is involved when learning to provide health care.[11]

Clearly, learners in the health professions need to do much of their practice in real clinical settings. However, much can also be done in small groups. Leaders can model and demonstrate highly relevant manual, intellectual, and communication skills, and learners can safely rehearse and refine these capabilities. For example, by inviting learners to role-play and to do various exercises (using such resources as paper-based cases, video triggers, and models and manikins), teachers can give learners increasing levels of challenge as they practice critical thinking, problem solving, physical assessment, various procedures,[12] active listening, advice giving, team building, and other necessary clinical skills. In addition, in all groups, even those not focused on developing explicit clinical skills, students can have opportunities to practice presenting ideas clearly, listening actively to each other, jointly addressing issues and problems, and other skills required of health professionals.

Learners can reflect on and assess experiences they've had inside and outside the group. Being reflective during and after experiences and regularly doing self-assessments of their capabilities are

---

[11]For further clarification of this process, you might find it helpful to reflect on your own learning of a complex skill outside of your profession, such as skiing, computing, or playing a musical instrument.

[12] In this book we do not focus explicitly on teaching manual skills. However, many of the issues in Chapter 8, "Teaching Communication Skills," are pertinent to the teaching of manual skills in groups.

vital activities for learners throughout their professional education and careers (Jason et al., 1978; Schön, 1983, 1987; Westberg & Jason, 1993, 1994b). Arthur Chickering (1977) argued that activities that are not checked by observation and analysis are often intellectual dead ends, leading neither to greater clarification nor to new ideas. Sports coaches routinely videotape and review their athletes' performance with them, recognizing that athletes, like all learners, need to intersperse review with their practice if they are to derive maximum learning from what they do. Even when learners are acquiring primarily cognitive material, David Kolb (1984) proposes that the ideal learning cycle proceeds from concrete experiences to observations and reflections, then to the formulation of abstract concepts and generalizations, and to testing the implications of these concepts in new situations. Donald Schön (1983) points out that professionals who become lifelong learners practice what he calls "reflection-in-action," the ability to reflect on one's thinking while acting. Phrases such as "thinking on your feet" suggest not only that we can think about what we've just done, we can think about what we're doing as we're doing it.[13]

To learn effectively during their professional education and throughout their careers, learners need to routinely reflect on what they are doing adequately and what still needs work. Becoming balanced and constructive in one's self-critiques takes practice and feedback from others.

Classroom and laboratory exercises, patient-care tasks, and projects in the community can provide learners with experiences that are rich in learning opportunities. However, learners are often under so much pressure to move quickly from one activity to another that much of the learning potential is often lost. In small groups, when there is trust between and among the facilitators and learners, experiences from outside the group can be reviewed safely and constructively. The learners can identify their strengths and areas needing further work, and they can get critique on their self-critique from their leader and peers (see Chapters 9 and 10). In addition, learners can reflect on and assess their experiences within the group, both while they are happening and afterward.

Reflection and self-assessment need to include attention to the emotional dimensions of experiences. Small groups can provide opportunities for giving appropriate and constructive attention to the human dimensions of learning and health care. When the emotional dimension of learning is neglected, as it is in some disciplines and programs in the health profes-

---

[13]For an instructional video on understanding and teaching this process, see Jason and colleagues 1978.

sions, learners can become practitioners who lack the emotional maturity to provide optimal whole person care to others. Learners who don't routinely reflect on the emotional impact of their experiences, whether while dissecting a cadaver, making a mistake while caring for a patient, or watching a patient die, may develop ways of dealing with their feelings that can be hurtful to themselves or others.

Learners can learn to ask for, provide, and use constructive feedback. Feedback is fundamental to learning. Learners need specific, accurate feedback on their performance, including what they are doing well and what still needs work. If they receive such feedback in a timely way, their learning is likely to be accelerated, their progress reinforced and sustained. Without feedback, learners' mistakes can go uncorrected, and they can develop and solidify bad habits. If they don't receive feedback on their strengths, they are at risk of discontinuing some of their desirable behaviors. For example, unless they receive feedback, learners who have instinctive skills as systematic problem solvers, or who are inherently sensitive to patients' concerns, or who have an effectively open-ended approach to interviewing, may not necessarily know they have these capabilities or that these capabilities are valued. Without reinforcement, these capabilities may be lost.

Feedback is not necessarily or automatically helpful. Improperly done, it can be hurtful. If learners receive harsh, insensitive feedback, they can develop a pattern of avoiding feedback, putting themselves at risk of diminished progress or sustained inadequacies. As we discuss in detail elsewhere (Westberg & Jason, 1991b, 1993, 1994a), to be helpful and constructive, feedback needs to be linked to actual observations of learners' performance, timely, descriptive of specific behaviors, presented in supportive, nonjudgmental ways, and when possible, tied to the learner's self-assessments.

Some group sessions are designed specifically to include opportunities for learners to ask for and get feedback. For example, in many skills development groups (e.g., groups that focus on the learning of interpersonal skills), following the learners' participation in role plays and other exercises, and their doing self-assessments, feedback is provided by the leader, group members, and any real or standardized patients who are involved (see Chapter 8). During discussions, learners can get feedback on their ideas and how they present them. In all groups there are opportunities for teachers and the learners' peers to provide learners with helpful feedback on their behaviors in the group, thus helping them enhance their effectiveness as communicators and team members, while also helping them learn the important skills of giving and receiving feedback.

Learners can have the time they need for meaningful learning. Much of our conventional teaching fails to acknowledge that lasting learning takes time. Little of value is learned in one pass. Repetition, reinforcement, and review are all needed for consolidating learning. In traditional lectures and conferences, the pace is set by teachers, most of whom do little or nothing to determine or adapt to the learning needs of the students. In fact, the typical pace is rushed as the teachers try to cram as much as they can into their allotted time, apparently not recognizing the limitations of uninterrupted verbal presentations. Some learners cannot assimilate spoken information well, most learners' attention diminishes over time, and few learners give their full attention to lectures for more than 10 minutes at a stretch (Stuart & Rutherford, 1978; Verner & Dickson, 1967).

In well-run groups, the facilitator is continuously checking on the learners' intellectual and emotional states, and ensuring that there are ample opportunities for questions and reviews. A central shift in mind-set and practice needed by teachers who are new to the small group setting is a readjustment of their sense and their management of time.

In small groups, students can learn from and with each other

Increasingly, scholars are impressed with what learners can contribute to their own and each other's learning (e.g., Johnson, Johnson, & Smith, 1991; Bruffee, 1993). And, as Abercrombie observed nearly two decades ago (1979) and many other educators have also concluded, students can learn some things more effectively in collaborative groups than on their own. The countless learners who have taken the initiative to form study groups appear to understand how helpful learners can be to each other. Some of the primary ways that learners can help each other in small groups are outlined next.

In groups, learners can broaden and enrich their individual and collective understandings and capabilities. Together they can build knowledge.[14] In health care, as in most profes-

---

[14] See Whitman (1993) for a discussion of "social constructivism," a theory that maintains that individuals use their membership in a community (group) to continually refine and shape their models of reality.

sions, there are multiple ways to view and approach most issues and problems. Yet, in many traditional lectures, learners are exposed to one dominant view—the teacher's. Because of their teachers' power in their lives, some learners uncritically accept their teachers' points of view and suspend their own thinking. In open, collaborative groups, however, learners are exposed to multiple perspectives, particularly if learners come from diverse backgrounds (ideally, as diverse as the people they will be working with and serving during their careers). Learners are also exposed to multiple approaches to people and problems, multiple ways of presenting ideas, expressing feelings, listening, and problem solving. This diversity can help learners clarify and stretch their understandings and capabilities.

In addition, collectively, group members can often achieve understandings and outcomes that are fuller and richer, even more accurate, than can be achieved by any of them individually with the same amount of time. Such groups are like well-functioning health teams (representing different perspectives and approaches) that are more effective than individual practitioners in understanding and helping patients with complex problems. In both situations, the team has more information collectively than any individual member, and the process of sharing what they know helps members expand their thinking and see in new ways. Another way of viewing collaborative knowledge building is the image of barn raising suggested by McCormick and Kahn (1986). Everyone's contribution can be helpful, and some of the building explicitly requires the cooperation of two or more people, or even the whole group, working as a unit.

Learners can sometimes be more effective than experts in helping each other learn. When traveling, many people recognize that to get accurate, helpful directions to a destination they should ask someone who recently made the trip successfully for the first time. They should not ask those who take that route frequently. Such people have typically come to do so automatically and are likely to have forgotten important details, such as a turn that needs to be made at a complex fork in the road. However, someone who has just struggled to get to that destination for the first time is likely to recall the details vividly and be able to provide appropriate warnings about potential problems.

A fuller way to conceptualize this issue is to think of how we make progress when becoming competent. This process can be thought of as occurring in the following four stages (adapted from *Personnel Journal*, 1974):

1. *Unconscious incompetence.* As beginners in an area, we typically don't know what can be known or done, or what we need to learn or do.
2. *Conscious incompetence.* Our initial progress in an area takes us to the point of recognizing some of what can be known or done, and we begin to identify some of our specific deficiencies.
3. *Conscious competence.* When we initially become competent in an area we can usually specify elements and sources of that competence.
4. *Unconscious competence.* After being competent in an area for some time we may lose conscious awareness of the elements and sources of our competence (like the person who has taken the same route to a destination for years).

Usually, educators are most effective when they are in Stage 3: conscious competence. Some faculty members make a continuous, special effort to remain in this stage so that they can be maximally helpful to their learners. Many faculty, however, advance to Stage 4; they become unconsciously competent. Their expertise in the areas they teach is so ingrained that they are no longer in touch with their own learning history. They no longer remember the steps they took in mastering the concepts or skills they teach, and they have forgotten the sources of difficulty or confusion they faced as beginners. On the other hand, learners who have only recently understood a difficult concept or mastered a skill are often in touch with the steps they took in getting there and know what might be especially helpful to others. In groups, for any given topic, the learners tend to be at various stages along this continuum, and there can be some at Stage 3 who can serve as helpful guides for their peers.

Students can learn by teaching. Many of us who teach find that preparing for and doing teaching can provide some of our best learning. In trying to explain concepts or demonstrate skills to others, we can become aware of holes in our thinking and uncertainties or inadequacies in our performance. If we are open and nondefensive, learners' questions can prompt us to look at material and tasks in fresh ways, get us to pay more attention to details and nuances, and, perhaps, revise our conclusions or approaches. The Johnson brothers (David and Roger) (1991) point out that the notion that we learn by interacting with others and teaching is hardly new. The Talmud states that to learn, one must have a learning partner. As early as the first century, Quintilian argued that students could benefit from teaching one another. Johann Amos Comenius (1592–1670) believed that students would benefit by teaching and being taught by other students.

Learners can support each other. The process of becoming a health professional can be stressful. This stress may be compounded by the hours students spend in large classes where it is difficult to establish relationships with other students or teachers and where a sense of competition among students is often fostered. Whether or not learners are supported by family, friends, or counselors, most can benefit from the sharing that can occur in trusting groups among people who are having similar experiences. In trust-based instructional groups, learners can be open about their anxieties, fears, frustrations, and hopes. They can recognize that they are not the only ones experiencing difficulties, and they can help each other face individual and common challenges (see Chapter 10).

Facilitating small groups can provide what we need for helping learners

We teach people, not subjects, or at least we should. Just as health care needs to be person-centered rather than condition- or disease-centered, so too education should be person-centered rather than subject-centered (Rogers, 1969). This doesn't mean that our subject matter is unimportant. It does mean that to facilitate meaningful learning of our subject matter or anything else, we need to know our learners as people and adapt what we do to their unique needs, backgrounds, and interests. To inspire and challenge students, to help them be active learners, to give them constructive feedback, we need to be guided by "diagnostic" information about them. We need access to what they already know and what they don't know, what they can and cannot do, what they care about and what they dislike. We need to be aware of their individual learning styles, how they think about and solve problems, how they interact with others, how they handle challenges, their personal values and priorities, and more. Gathering some of this information directly from learners gives us access to the important, additional dimension of their self-perceptions. Also, since providing health care involves overt practice, since it is a performing art, we need to witness learners in action; we must observe them learning and doing professional tasks. Without such diagnostic information we can't have accurate or complete estimates of their actual capabilities and are unlikely to be optimally helpful.

Gathering this information, however, is not always easy or straight-forward. Diagnostic information gathering, in teaching as in health care, requires a relationship based on trust. In health care, we must earn patients' trust before they are likely to reveal their private worries and vulnerabilities. In education, before learners are likely to be fully open—to reveal their uncertainties, concerns, fears, and problems—with us and their peers, they must trust us and feel that we will use what we learn about them only in their best interests.

When teaching in a traditional lecture format, it is difficult to get to know learners at a meaningful level, to gather the diagnostic information about them that we need, or to establish the trust required for them to be fully candid. Individual learners just can't have enough airtime to reveal much about themselves or to get to know each other. Even if we've managed to get to know our students in other settings, during lectures it's not possible to be responsive to their individual needs and interests. However, in small groups, particularly those we meet with multiple times, it is relatively easier to get to know our learners as people and to establish caring, trust-based relationships. Indeed, as we've indicated, trust must be developed if small groups are to fulfill their potential.

Also, in traditional lectures there are not adequate opportunities to see learners in action. In groups, however, we can observe learners as they engage in tasks that are central to being a health professional: presenting and clarifying information and arguments, questioning other students and us, expressing feelings, approaching and solving problems, and much more. If we invite them to engage in role plays and other exercises that pertain to the real tasks of being health professionals, we can get important clues as to how they handle themselves in real life situations. If group members reflect aloud on their actions and experiences within and outside the group, we can get some sense of how they perceive and assess themselves and each other.

In large groups, it is not always possible to detect students who need special help or who have unrecognized strengths, particularly if they are not active participants. In interactive small groups, where all students are encouraged to participate and it's not possible to hide, we are more likely to spot learners with special needs or unusual strengths. In such groups, if we are alert, we can identify students who, despite acceptable or even high grades on examinations, aren't able to apply their acquired information to systematic reasoning or problem solving. Conversely, we can identify students who are not doing well on conventional examinations but who demonstrate a good grasp of the material and good reasoning ability when confronting lifelike issues in small groups. Since participating in small groups requires the use of interpersonal communication skills, groups are a particularly good place to identify learners with special gifts or problems in this area.

Interacting with learners in small groups can bring important additional advantages: the experience can be stimulating and renewing for us. As Christensen (1991, p. 18) put it, "By bringing unexpected points of view and creative, upsetting questions to material that has become extremely familiar to the instructor, fresh and energetic students play a particularly useful role in class: they wake us up."

There can be positive spin-offs from small group learning

The tasks in which students engage while learning (e.g., listening and note-taking in traditional lectures; interacting with peers, negotiating decisions in small groups) can have a considerable impact on learners beyond the stated goals of these classes. The instructional process itself can affect how they behave as learners in other classes during their professional education and how they learn, teach, and practice during their careers.

Students who spend many hours in lectures, being essentially passive and subservient, are at risk of becoming or remaining passive, dependent learners who have little or no confidence in their capacities for self-directed learning. They may even be unaware that they need to be active learners. The impact of this process can be substantial and long lasting; often longer lasting than the information conveyed in this setting. Learners may become unwilling or unable to take initiative in pursuing their own learning. They may come to believe that passive exposure to other people's presentations is sufficient for their learning. They may be insufficiently critical of the noninteractive, marginally relevant presentations to which they are often exposed at continuing education meetings. Some of these learners may become teachers who perpetuate the lecture tradition. In addition, learners who are educated primarily in this authoritarian model may, in turn, treat patients in authoritarian ways (Westberg & Jason, 1993). Further, learners who do not have opportunities to learn from and with peers are not likely to be adequately equipped to pursue peer learning or to provide health care in partnership with others. Such outcomes can be highly undesirable given that high-quality health care increasingly requires teamwork within and among disciplines and professions. Such negative spin-offs of instruction are hardly anyone's explicit intention, and not all students are affected in the same ways, but the potential consequences are sufficiently serious that they deserve our reflection and careful attention.

In contrast, students who spend significant time as active learners in small groups are likely to begin feeling responsible for their learning generally and to have a balanced sense of confidence in their own views, together with an awareness of their need to be open to and reflect on the views of others. Such learners are likely to have developed the skills they need for directing their own learning (e.g., the ability to identify their learning needs, to develop learning goals and strategies) and to use these skills in other courses and throughout their careers. In other courses and later in continuing education programs, these students are more likely to challenge experiences in which they are expected to be passive. They are likely to seek out opportunities to be active learners. In addition, because they have been invited to be partners in their learning, they are more likely to generalize from this experience and invite patients to work with them as partners in their health care.

Further, learners who have had opportunities to learn from and with peers are likely to seek out more such opportunities. For example, as practitioners they might form study groups with colleagues. They might also be better equipped to benefit from consultations with colleagues than can their peers who didn't have practice learning effectively with others. As practitioners, students who worked and learned in groups are also more likely to have developed the attitudes and capabilities needed for working effectively on teams (e.g., they are able to value different perspectives and capabilities, identify and use the strengths of others, do joint planning and problem-solving, negotiate conflicts, and more). In other words, the experiences of working and learning collaboratively with peers can prepare them for working and learning with colleagues in the real world.

In summary, borrowing the provocative title of Marshall McLuhan's influential book (1967), *The Medium is the Message*, the communication processes in which we engage can have consequences beyond the content they convey and beyond their intentions. Regardless of the information or skills dealt with, the act of sitting in a traditional lecture can have an impact on learners that is different from (and less desirable than) the impact of the experience of being in a collaborative, interactive small group.

In interviews we've done at institutions with two-track systems, we've been told by clinical educators that they can spot which students were in the small-group track during their initial education and which were in the lecture-based track. After seeing patients, the small-group learners, without being told to do so, tend to study about the conditions they encountered and the next day seek to discuss what they learned with their instructors. In contrast, the lecture-track students seldom take such initiative and, in addition, often label their counterparts as "apple polishers." In seeking to demean the mature learning styles of their classmates, these learners are unintentionally revealing their view that learning is done to please one's teachers, not for one's own professional growth. Such students, unfortunately, are damaged learners. The system has not served them well.

COLLABORATION: AN ESSENTIAL CHARACTERISTIC OF EFFECTIVE GROUPS

The reasons that we just presented for using small groups in health professions education suggest what is possible, not what necessarily occurs whenever a teacher and a group of students meet. Securing the active participation of learners and helping them become competent clinicians is most likely to occur in groups based on a collaborative approach to learning. Here we examine the collaborative approach. In the next section we discuss some other characteristics of effective groups.

The collaborative approach can perhaps be explained best by contrasting it with the authoritarian approach.[15] In brief, in the collaborative model students are active participants in their learning; in the authoritarian model, learners are recipients of their teachers' decisions and actions. If you observe a small group in which the teacher uses a collaborative approach, you are likely to see learners engaged with each other and with the tasks at hand. If you observe a group in which the teacher uses an authoritarian approach, it will look much like a lecture class, only with fewer students. The teacher will probably be talking; the learners will be sitting passively, perhaps listening, perhaps daydreaming. When authoritarian educators do raise or invite questions, they typically interact with learners one at a time rather than engaging the whole group.

In Table 1.1 (p. 20) we summarize the contrasting characteristics of "pure" collaborative and authoritarian small groups. Most instructional

---

[15] To at least some extent, teachers need to be authoritative. The term authoritative describes their level of competence in their discipline; authoritarian describes their relationship style.

Table 1.1 Collaborative and Authoritarian Small Groups

	Collaborative	*Authoritarian*
Description of group	Learning community	Isolated individuals
Way learners are viewed	Vital contributors to their own and each other's learning	Recipients of teaching
Teacher's main roles	Facilitator of learning, Diagnostician, Model, Coach	Purveyor of information
Teacher's main communication	Questioning, Active listening	Telling
Type of leadership	Situational: varies with the learners and the context	Directive
Learners' main roles	*Active*: Questioners, Intent listeners, Discoverers, Teachers of each other	*Passive*: Listeners, Receivers of information, Note-takers
Nature of discussions	Dialogues; Reflective	Monologues
Nature of relationships	Trusting, Respectful, Collaborative	Formal, Guarded, Distant, Competitive, perhaps Adversarial
Responsibility for sessions	Increasingly, the learners'	The teacher's

groups in the health professions are something of a mixture. They do not fit exclusively into either of these categories.

Collaborative and authoritarian educators differ greatly in their assumptions about learners and learning.[16] Collaborative educators make the kinds of assumptions we described in the first part of the chapter. They anticipate that students and residents are likely to have understandings, experiences, skills, feelings, and interests that are relevant to the learning goals and that they can examine and build on this foundation. They assume that learners can make helpful contributions to the group process and can build knowledge together. (In fact, collaborative leaders often find they

---

[16] Some teachers function out of habit, without reflecting on or articulating, or even being aware of their underlying assumptions. However, their assumptions can be inferred from their behavior. As Chris Argyris (1982) points out, people don't always behave congruently with their espoused theories (what they say), but they do behave congruently with their "theories-in-use," their "mental models."

learn from their students.) Because collaborative educators think it is essential for students to do their own learning and be active, skilled learners, they see their main roles as guiding and facilitating learning, primarily by being diagnostic (determining what learners need and want); modeling capabilities learners need to develop; and coaching learners as they try to do things for themselves. Authoritarian teachers, on the other hand, treat learners as if they were vessels to be filled. They see their job as conveying to learners what they need to know and the students' jobs as listening and absorbing.

Collaborative educators use a situational style of leadership. The extent to which they are directive or facilitative depends on their assessment of such factors as the learners' competence and confidence with their learning tasks and with the group's developmental stage. For example, when a group is meeting for the first time and learning a new task, the educator might determine that the learners need guidance, so initially she might be directive, but in a way that helps students learn quickly to do things for themselves. As learners are ready, she typically shifts to the role of coach — raising questions, encouraging self-assessment, and providing feedback. Finally, as learners are able to work independently, the educator fades into the background, delegating but not abdicating responsibility. This cycle of modeling, coaching, and fading (Collins, Brown, & Newman, 1989) to which we have added the key initial step of diagnosing/assessing, occurs with each new significant task so at the same session the leader might play several roles (e.g., model a new task, coach learners as they independently do another task; see Figure 1.1).[17] In contrast, authoritarian educators are directive most of the time. They tend not to be diagnostic and they tend to treat most learners and small groups in the same way.

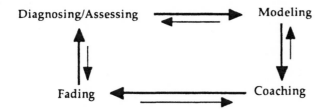

Figure 1.1 Cyclical leadership roles in small groups.

---

[17] The figure indicates that in teaching new skills the leader may need to return to an earlier stage (e.g., move back from coaching to modeling, if learners don't appear to have an adequate picture of the skill). We deal with this and other issues in Chapter 2.

Collaborative educators try to help their groups become communities of learners instead of gatherings of isolated individuals. Christensen (1991) suggests that in "learning communities" diverse backgrounds blend and individuals bond into an association dedicated to collective as well as personal learning. Particularly as groups spend extended time together there is a sense of collective and personal belonging that may be expressed in "we" language, in joking and laughter. Learners may change seats at successive sessions so they can sit next to different group members. Learners may arrive early and leave late in an effort to spend more time together (Jones, Barnlund, & Haiman, 1980). Mutual trust makes it possible for learners to take the kinds of risks (e.g., venturing opinions, asking questions) often needed for significant learning. Whether learners are discovering new concepts, solving problems, or questioning factual information, Slavin and colleagues (1985) reported that a collaborative approach helps them gain self-esteem and develop academic skills while also promoting understanding of the subject matter.

In a group dominated by an authoritarian approach, learners are likely to be careful to avoid exposing their shortcomings. In addition, they may lack confidence in their own thinking and conclusions. Symptoms of competition are common (e.g., students rushing to be the first to answer questions, demeaning what other students say or do as a way of trying to elevate themselves, using humor at other students' expense).[18]

---

[18] For this discussion of collaborative and authoritarian leadership we acknowledge our debt to Kurt Lewin (1948), a pioneer in the study of groups. He identified three styles of leadership: *autocratic*, *democratic*, and *laissez-faire*. The way he and others describe the autocratic model is similar to our description of authoritarian leadership (e.g., autocratic leaders make virtually all of the group's decisions; autocratic groups are leader-centered). The democratic model is similar to our collaborative model. Democratic leaders work with the group in developing plans that are agreeable to everyone; their statements are intended to guide rather than to direct, and they give their expert information only when it is pertinent, not in an effort to gain status. Democratic leaders support spontaneous shifts in direction and methods that emerge from within the group and that all agree are within the limits defined by the group. Democratic groups are member-centered (Sampson & Marthas, 1977). In the laissez-faire model, leaders abdicate power. They don't attempt to engage learners in conversation or involve them in other ways. They simply leave things alone to develop as they will.

Our decision to use the terms *authoritarian* and *collaborative* to characterize small group leadership was made in part because we have used these terms extensively in earlier writing about clinical supervision and see the processes as fully parallel. Also, for us, unlike the autocratic or democratic leader who each have one particular way of functioning, the collaborative leader exercises different levels of power and directiveness depending on the circumstances and the needs of the group members. (As Hersey and Blanchard pointed out (1969), effective leadership isn't either autocratic or democratic, it is "situational".) See Chapter 2 for a discussion of leadership.

ADDITIONAL CHARACTERISTICS OF EFFECTIVE INSTRUCTIONAL GROUPS

Our observations of small groups, our direct work with groups, our experiences as faculty developers with health professions educators who facilitate small groups, and our review of the literature have led us to conclude that small groups in health professions education are most likely to achieve their potential if, in addition to being collaborative, they have the characteristics discussed below. Not all these characteristics are likely to be evident the first time a group meets. Effective groups take time to develop. These characteristics are goals toward which group facilitators and members can strive.

The teacher is comfortable being a group leader and has the necessary skills. Significant factors in determining the effectiveness of instructional groups are the leader's personal characteristics (including personality) and skill level. Teachers are usually in a position of considerable power. They can make or break the group experience. Their needs for power and control, or their comfort relinquishing it as the learners are ready, can be major components in determining a group's success. In Chapter 3, we discuss the influence of teachers' personal characteristics and capabilities on the group process.

Members respect and trust each other. Mutual respect and trust are essential ingredients of effective groups. They make it possible for teachers and students to be open and honest with each other. Mutual trust implies that all members of the group are respectful of whatever is revealed to them—particularly personal vulnerabilities and other intimate information about group members—and they do not use what they learn to hurt group members or anyone else. If learners are to take the kinds of risks required for significant learning, such as being open about their strengths and weaknesses and being willing to go through the awkward periods that inevitably accompany the learning of new attitudes and complex skills, they need to feel they can fully trust every member of the group, including the teacher.

The group's size is conducive to everyone's active participation. There is no single optimal size for instructional small groups. The appropriate size depends on such factors as the nature of the tasks to be done, the amount of time available, and the skills of the leader. We discuss the important issue of group size in Chapter 2.

Group membership is reasonably stable.   In effective groups, members attend regularly and arrive on time. Groups that are continually losing and replacing members squander time orienting the new members and relearning how to work together (Schwarz, 1994). When members attend irregularly or are late to sessions, the process is disrupted. (Some task-dominated groups, such as morning work rounds in clinical settings, often have a continuously changing membership. Unless all members have solid relationships from other settings or long-standing colleagueship, such groups may get some tasks done reasonably well, but the learning potential is typically less than it might otherwise be.)

Learners have a common sense of direction and purpose. Effective instructional groups have general, overall purposes (e.g., develop problem-solving skills or communication skills, provide support) and shared learning goals that are understood and accepted by all members. (In part, a group can be distinguished from a collection of individuals by its common goals.) Some or all of the learning goals may be established by the faculty member or the institution in advance of the group sessions. In other situations learners generate some or all of their goals or they have opportunities to modify and refine the goals presented by the faculty. The goals might be fairly specific (e.g., the group is expected to refine the hypothesis-generation skills they use while solving clinical problems), or they might be nonspecific (e.g., students are to explore their feelings about caring for dying patients). Even if the goals are specific, learners are not rigidly tied to them. For example, if unexpected events reveal compelling needs or interests, the group might decide to create new goals and even modify existing ones. Regardless of how the goals are developed or how specific they are, members feel a shared ownership of them.

Learners also accept and feel ownership of their ways of working together.   In effective instructional groups, learners typically are involved in deciding how they will work together and feel ownership of the decisions that are made. All groups develop norms that are implicit or explicit. In effective groups, members make these norms explicit, often calling them ground rules.

David Johnson (1970) says that for group norms to be effective, members must recognize they exist (make them explicit), feel some internal commitment to them, and observe that other group members accept and follow them. He says that members are most likely to develop ownership of ground rules if they see them as useful in accomplishing the goals and tasks to which they are committed. Factors that help determine whether members will conform to the group norms, according to Beebe and Masterson (1993), are the personalities of the group members, the clarity of the norms and the certainty of consequences for breaking them, the number of people who have broken the norms, the quality of relationships among group members, and the sense of group identification.

Learners are clear about their roles and responsibilities. Unless a purpose of the group is for learners to work on identifying their roles and responsibilities, groups usually make the most progress when they address these issues early and directly. Roles and responsibilities can change, so they may need to be revisited.

Learners feel responsible for the group and for each other. In well-functioning groups, members contribute to the group's activities and try to ensure that everyone can participate. If members think that something isn't working, they don't just wait for the leader to notice what's wrong and fix it. Rather, they speak up and do what they can to help the group accomplish its goals.

The group recognizes and deals constructively with conflict. Since individuals each create their own views of reality, group members may have different—even conflicting—views and values. Effective groups recognize and welcome differences that are expressed in constructive ways, appreciating that differences can stimulate members to examine their assumptions, helping them stretch and enrich their thinking, individually and collectively.

Early in the life of a group, members are likely to hold back irritations, frustrations, and strong personal opinions. As intimacy and trust develop or as learners feel pressure to accomplish group tasks, members are likely to become more candid, even aggressively assertive. At this stage, heated conflict may emerge. Effective groups handle such conflict constructively. Indeed one of the signs that a group is cohesive and that members have a strong bond is the group's ability to tolerate and manage conflict (Bormann, 1989). In a highly cohesive group, members know they will not be rejected for their views and, therefore, are willing to express them even though such expression may provoke disagreement. In contrast, some groups get stuck at earlier stages of group development. They may avoid conflict and even fall into *groupthink* (Janis, 1972), a pattern of avoiding conflict and adopting an approach in which "good group members" show their loyalty to the group's leader and other members by never really challenging or seriously doubting the leader's or the group's wisdom in matters of decision making.[19]

Susan Wheelan (1990, p. 19) contends that "conflict is necessary for the establishment of a safe environment."

> While this may, at first glance, seem paradoxical, conflict is helpful to the development of trust. We know, from our own experience, that it is easier to develop trust in another person or in a group if we believe that we can disagree and we won't be abandoned or hurt for our difference. It is difficult to trust those who deny us the right to be ourselves. . . . To engage in conflict with others and to work it out is an exhilarating experience. It provides energy, a commonly shared experience, a sense of safety and authenticity, and allows for deeper intimacy and collaboration. . . .. We also know from experience that conflict can lead to the destruction of relationships. Many groups get stuck in this stage and cannot progress. . . .. Thus while this stage cannot be avoided since it is the only route to mature collaboration, most of us would rather avoid the conflict stage in group development. As with individual development, however, groups that avoid this stage remain dependent, insecure, and incapable of true collaboration and productive work.

The group monitors its progress.   Productive groups keep their goals in sight and monitor whether they are staying on track, while recognizing that groups sometimes go off on tangents that can be useful and meaningful. Group members are aware of what they are doing and explicitly decide whether and when they want to alter their game plan.

Group members can have fun.   In many effective groups, laughter can often be heard. Although members of well-functioning groups take learning seriously, they often retain a capacity for playfulness, allowing for flights of fancy and for refreshing moments of respite from their work. In such groups, members can appreciate, even laugh at, incongruities, inconsistencies, and other irregularities. Light fun that is not at anyone's expense can also ease conflicts and disagreements. Meaningful learning, which requires that learners make changes in how they think and function, can be hard work, even painful. Making progress and fulfilling worthy goals, however, can provide a genuine sense of accomplishment. They deserve to be enjoyed and celebrated.

---

[19] For discussions of stages in group evolution and approaches to managing conflict, see Chapter 4.

Over time, teachers may reduce their active involvement in their groups. Typically, when groups first start meeting, teachers need to be fairly active, doing such things as establishing a trusting climate determining the learners' goals and expectations, clarifying any goals that the program might have for them, helping learners establish some of their own goals, forming impressions of the learners' levels of readiness, and helping the learners select experiences and strategies that are likely to be appropriate for achieving their goals. Over time, as the students become more active in their learning and take increasing responsibility for the work of the group, the faculty member retreats further into the background. Some teachers may even skip some sessions.

Healthy groups are like healthy families. The characteristics of effective and ineffective groups can be understood, in part, by their parallels to healthy and dysfunctional families. We summarize these parallels in Table 1.2. Significant learning and personal growth are much more likely in healthy groups and families.

Table 1.2 Characteristics of healthy and dysfunctional groups and families

Healthy groups/families	*Dysfunctional groups/families*
Respect for feelings/ thoughts of others	Feelings/thoughts of others are ignored/demeaned
Individual differences are encouraged	Conformity is expected
Open communication predominates	Members have secrets
Dynamic, changing, flowing	Static, rigid
Decisions are reached after discussion	Decisions are made unilaterally or repeatedly deferred
Self-imposed, flexible rules	Rigid rules imposed by tradition or an individual
Open discussion of problems	Denial of problems
Assertion, empathy, grace	Aggression, codependency, despair
Feel empowered	Feel victimized

SUMMARY

Preparing health professionals who will be highly competent and who will continue to learn throughout their careers is a daunting challenge. Collaborative, interactive small groups provide the opportunities and conditions that can enable us to meet much of that challenge. In small groups, students can learn from and with each other, and we can provide what is needed for worthy, lasting learning. In addition, as facilitators of small learning groups we can have access to much of what we need for being optimally helpful to learners. And there can be positive spin-offs from small group learning. For example, learners are likely to become and remain self-directed and effective in learning from and with their colleagues. Being collaborative learners during their basic professional education can even help prepare learners for being collaborative later with colleagues and patients.

Securing all these many benefits from teaching and learning in the small group setting is contingent, in large part, on using a collaborative, not an authoritarian, instructional approach and on several other conditions. The teachers must be comfortable as group leaders and have the necessary skills. Emphasis needs to be on mutual respect and trust, and group membership should be reasonably stable. Also, the learners need to have a sense of direction and purpose, feel a genuine sense of "ownership" of the goals, be clear about their roles and responsibilities, feel responsible for the group and for each other, have adequate opportunities to participate, explicitly agree upon reasonable ground rules for working together, and recognize and deal with conflict constructively. Further, learning is most likely to be successful if the learners enjoy what they are doing.

CHAPTER 2

Preparing for Leading Small Groups

Students and residents do not automatically learn the information and skills they need when meeting in small groups. When learning experiences have not been carefully planned, learners can be frustrated and come away having not learned much. Or, worse yet, some experiences can be what John Dewey called "mis-educative" (1938), they may arrest or distort the growth of further learning or take the learners in undesirable directions.

A teacher who agrees to lead a small group but does insufficient preparation may face difficulties at the first group session. For example, if a teacher fails to find out in advance about the learners' current capabilities, the learning goals and activities that he plans might be too elementary or too advanced for the learners. Or if she fails to identify and arrange for the equipment and materials needed during the session, a leader might not have what she needs to do what she intended.

Some teachers know what they need to do to prepare for sessions but do not take the time required for attending to these tasks. Other teachers are not aware of their available choices or of the likely impact of each choice and so don't take action or aren't in a position to make good decisions. For example, if a group leader is not aware that a quiet room with appropriately arranged furniture can be important to a session's success, he might not bother to check out or arrange the room in advance. Even if he arrives at the room before the session is to start and the room arrangement is suboptimal, he is likely to leave it that way if he is not aware that some room arrangements can adversely affect the learning experience.

To ensure that small group sessions are worthwhile and not mis-educative, to avoid unwelcome surprises, and to help prevent other problems from occurring, we recommend attending to a number of tasks prior to the first session. These preparatory tasks include gathering the information needed for planning effective learning experiences or for reviewing the plans made by others (e.g., the course coordinator). These tasks include making or reviewing decisions that are often overlooked or made by default.

You might attend to the tasks and decisions described in this chapter alone or with others, including the learners.[1] If the group you will be conducting is part of a larger course, and the course coordinator has attended to some tasks and decisions that will have an impact on you and your group, be sure that you can accept these decisions. If not, we suggest doing what you can to help improve what is planned for your group.

Although there is some order to the way we present the following tasks and decisions, they are not fully sequential or neatly linear and are not in priority sequence.

Determining or clarifying the group's size and mix of characteristics

Although you may not have control over which or how many learners join your group, the following are two issues to consider if you do.

Group size.   Because groups need to be small enough so that all learners can participate, a key question is how many students can actively participate in the intended activities? For example, many agree that the optimal size for most problem-based learning groups (Chapter 7) is roughly five to eight members, but more students can participate actively in other kinds of groups. Remember, as group size increases, the complexity of the interrelationships in the group can increase exponentially, not just arithmetically, and it can become difficult for learners to have sufficient opportunity for meaningful participation.[2] On the other hand, if the group size is

---

[1] Being involved in planning their group sessions can contribute to the learners' sense of ownership of their learning. Tapping into their knowledge of the group members' needs and interests can enhance the sessions.

[2] Authoritarian leaders may not perceive any problem with increased group sizes. In didactic groups, the number of learners present—even their characteristics—make little difference, since most of what happens is teacher-centered and teacher-controlled and is largely independent of the learners. Of course, the price of the seeming tranquility in such groups is diminished meaningful, lasting learning.

too small, there might be insufficient diversity of ideas or too few people for the tasks that need to be accomplished. If some of the intended group activities are best suited for a relatively larger number of learners and others are better with fewer learners, the group can be temporarily divided into subgroups (e.g., of twos or threes) for these latter activities.

Group mix. Most group experiences are enriched (although, perhaps, made initially more difficult to manage) if the members are from different age groups and diverse cultural and educational backgrounds. Having members from different disciplines can also be useful. The learning goals for the group sessions should determine the extent to which the group should be heterogeneous. If, for example, the learners are preparing for working on interdisciplinary health teams, the group membership should include representatives from the health professions that will be on those future teams. In general, it's best if learners are at similar levels of proficiency.

Discovering who the learners are

As we discussed in Chapter 1, to plan group experiences that will be maximally helpful to learners, we need to know them as people, and we need information on their prior experiences and current learning needs. Ideally you will be able to begin getting to know the learners prior to the group session (e.g., by talking with them individually, by having them fill out questionnaires). Whether or not advance information gathering is possible, it's also important, as we discuss in Chapter 4, to work at getting to know your learners during the group sessions.

Determining or clarifying where the group experience fits into the overall curriculum

If you are involved in deciding where the group sessions will fit into the curriculum, try to ensure that they build on, integrate sequentially into, and support the overall learning goals of the curriculum. If the learners are from different disciplines or at different levels in their education, integrating with multiple curricula will clearly take some effort, but doing so will likely be rewarded with a more valuable learning experience. Even if you will not be involved in these decisions, at least be aware of experiences the learners have had prior to, and are having concurrently with, your group sessions. These other experiences will likely have an impact on your group. In working on this curricular integration, consider the following questions.

What experiences have the group members had with the topic(s) and capabilities(s) that are to be addressed? If during other courses learners have dealt with the topic(s) and capabilities(s) intended for your group, find out what their prior experiences have been so that you can plan how to provide them with an appropriate level of challenge. Consider asking faculty members who have previously addressed your subject areas with these learners how they think you can build on what has already been done. If you have advance access to some of the students, ask them what they feel they have learned and what they still need to learn in the areas of your concern. Also, consider planning some activities for your first meeting that will give you additional "diagnostic" information about their levels of readiness.

What have been the learners' experiences with the kind of group you intend to lead? If during their time at your institution these learners have never participated in a learning group or in the specific kind of group you will be offering (e.g., a problem-based learning group), at your first meeting with the group you may need to be prepared to help them understand the rationale for what they will be doing. If they have had relevant group experiences, it is important to find out how they regarded those experiences and, if necessary, to try overcoming problems they may have encountered.

To what extent are they accustomed to being active learners? If the learners in your group are accustomed to being passive, you will probably need to help them understand and value active learning and develop the skills they need as active learners. If your instructional approach will be a departure from the dominant pattern in your program, be prepared for the possibility that some or many learners will resist adapting to this new way of functioning. Even if they understand that there are merits to active learning, people who feel stretched to their limits (as do many learners in the health professions) have little residual energy for modifying their ways of functioning. If many students resist your efforts to have them become more active learners, you may need to try influencing the overall educational climate at your institution. If your institution is trying to help all students be more active in their learning, you might suggest that the faculty hold sessions for incoming students on why and how to be active learners.

Is the group freestanding or part of a larger course or other activity? Some groups are part of larger courses (e.g., in the small groups students discuss topics introduced in prior lectures). Some are tied to clinical experiences (e.g., students meet weekly to discuss the patients they've been seeing). Some groups are freestanding (e.g., a monthly support group in which the learners talk about any topic they choose). If your group is not freestanding and you are not adequately familiar with the course or activity to which it is linked, you will probably need to learn what you can about the goals, instructional atmosphere, and relationship styles of that umbrella activity. Also, if one of the purposes of your group sessions is enabling learners to reflect on events that are external to the group (e.g., interactions with patients, a panel discussion), try to arrange for the group sessions to be held as soon after those other events as possible so they will still be fresh in the learners' minds.

How much time will be devoted to the group sessions, and how will that time be distributed? If you are involved in deciding how many times the group will meet and how long each session should be, consider how much time is needed for successfully achieving the purposes for which the group is being created. If a goal is for the learners to learn to work together effectively, remember that it can take many meetings before members are likely to function as an effective team.[3]

The amount of time scheduled for group sessions and the way the time is distributed can affect how you plan for the session(s), when you do your planning, and the focus of your planning. If you have only a single, relatively brief session (under 2 hours), virtually all your planning needs to be done ahead of time, and your focus is likely to be limited. With a group that meets only once, you may not be able to devote much time to group process issues. On the other hand, with a group that meets multiple times, you can do some planning prior to each meeting, and you will likely need to spend time on group process issues, even if your goals are primarily task-oriented.

What activities will be concurrent with your group sessions? The amount of energy and time that students devote to groups can be influenced by their concurrent commitments. If possible, don't schedule group sessions when learners need to devote substantial time and thought to preparing for exams or other time-consuming activities.

---

[3] In some clinical settings, the composition of the group that reviews patients changes daily. If you want learners to enjoy some of the values of small group learning described in Chapter 1, we recommend trying to work out strategies so that learners can be together in the same group on multiple occasions.

Determining or clarifying the overall purpose and the learning goals

As we discussed in Chapter 1, we and our learners need a sense of general direction, even if we don't know precisely where we'll end up. Formulating goals involves setting priorities and making choices among potential areas of emphasis so that the group will make best use of its time. Goals can also provide the framework for monitoring the learners' progress, individually and as a group. Of course, whether overtly articulated or not, goals are always set. When not set in advance or with care, they are set accidentally or by default, neither of which is likely to provide the sense of direction learners need or ensure that the eventual outcomes are desirable. In some courses the only articulated evidence of the teachers' real expectations is the final exam, which is both unfair and educationally useless. Here we discuss *preformulated goals* (goals that are typically developed by the faculty prior to the first group session). In Chapter 4, we discuss goals that are developed jointly with learners, usually during the initial group sessions. Whether you were involved in developing the goals or you are reviewing goals developed by others, consider reflecting on the following questions.

Are the goals sufficiently specific?   As we discussed in Chapter 1, goals can range from specific to nonspecific. Nonspecific goals are useful for the open-ended exploration learners might engage in during some discussion groups. However, if learners are expected to develop specific skills by the end of the session(s) (e.g., be able to do a complete sexual history), these expectations need to be explicit.

Are the goals clear and understandable?   Goals are often cryptic summaries of considerable prior thought and discussion. They are best understood by those who developed them. To be useful, goals need to be understood by all involved faculty members and learners. So, if possible, both groups should participate in developing or refining the goals. If the goals were developed by others, be sure you understand their full implications and can explain them to your learners.

Are the goals appropriate for the learners' stages of development?   Instructors who are experts in a field may have lost touch with what is appropriate for beginners or even for moderately advanced learners. As previously discussed, they may be unconsciously competent. To ensure the appropriateness of goals, have them reviewed by faculty and/or students who are familiar with the learners' current stage of development.

Can the goals be achieved with the available resources and the time allotted? Advance planning should include developing a rough estimate of the amount of time and the physical and human resources that are likely to be needed for achieving the group's goals. If adjustments will be needed, you and your learners will be far better off if this discovery is made before it is too late to do anything constructive about any mismatch.

Are the goals worthwhile? Have the most worthwhile goals been defined? In general, it is easier to write goals and specific objectives for technical skills (e.g., examining and cleaning a surgical incision) than for interpersonal skills (e.g., the capacity to demonstrate empathy) or attitudes (e.g., a sense of responsibility for one's own learning). Be sure that complex, hard-to-describe goals are not overlooked just because they are harder (or even impossible) to define with precision. Also be sure the goals are relevant for your learners' actual careers (e.g., some goals in some basic science courses are not relevant to future clinicians).

Are the goals consistent with the overall goals of the school or program? Ideally, schools and graduate programs have a written list of key competencies that learners need to develop before graduating from the program. If these overall goals are worthy and achievable, ensure that the goals for your group sessions are consistent with and supportive of these program goals.

Are the goals considered modifiable and dynamic? Some goals may be nonnegotiable. For example, you and other faculty members might decide that by the end of the group sessions you expect all of the learners to be able to demonstrate during a role play that they can take a complete health history. This dominant goal may be the basis for the entire course and not subject to modification. However, there may be many other goals that could be adjustable, depending on the events that emerge during the evolution of the group. Leaving yourselves as open as possible enables the group to take advantage of unexpected learning opportunities.

Should the goals and objectives be in writing? Generally, the answer is an emphatic "yes." A written document ensures that all teachers and learners have the same basic information. When core goals for a course are not in writing, there is a risk that they will be significantly altered as different teachers impose their interpretive twists while conveying them to their groups. Typically the very process of putting goals in writing leads to clearer, better statements: inconsistencies, contradictions and ambiguities are more likely to be recognized and corrected.

Will learners be developing goals? If students are to become self-directed learners, they need practice in setting and pursuing their own learning goals. They are most likely to become skilled at setting goals and to appreciate the importance of their doing so if most teachers expect this of them. If you are the first to set this expectation, your request may be met with bewilderment, even resistance. As we've indicated, learners often oppose efforts to get them to function in unfamiliar ways.

Determining or clarifying the group learning activities

When groups meet for the first time, typical opening activities include introductions, an orientation, and a discussion about how best to work together (see Chapter 4). Most of the session is devoted to one or more explicit learning activities. As you plan the learning activities or review plans others have made, consider the following questions.

Are the activities supportive of and consistent with the learning goals? Clearly, whatever activities you plan should be an outgrowth of and consistent with the goals for the group. If the process of planning the activities reveals that the goals are incomplete or inadequate, they should be changed.

Will the activities be undertaken within an appropriate context? Abstract discussions or exercises that learners view as irrelevant are likely to fall flat. Learners are likely to feel most motivated to engage in those group activities they feel are linked to the challenges they are having or anticipate facing in the real world. For example, students are most likely to be motivated to learn about the anatomy and physiology of the human body if their exploration is linked to a patient case or problem. Learners are also most likely to later retrieve and use what they've learned if their learning occurs in the context of considering real-world situations.

Will the context for the group's activities be provided by external or internal experiences, or both? John Dewey and Jean Piaget were among those who contributed to our understand of the centrality of experience in learning. Eduard C. Lindeman (1926, pp. 9–10), a pioneer in adult education, observed that "the resource of highest value in adult education is the learner's experience. . . . Too much of learning consists of vicarious substitution of someone else's experience and knowledge." Once learners begin observing and participating in real-world professional activities,[4] their own experiences will provide the basis for some of their most meaningful learning. In Chapter 9 we discuss how group sessions can be built around helping learners reflect on their care of patients. External experiences can also be stories the learners read (e.g., an account of a person's experience with a chronic illness) or large group, patient-focused presentations they attend.

During group sessions you can also create shared experiences that provide a context for learning.[5] For example, you can give learners a real-world problem to solve as a context for refining their skills as problem solvers or for reflecting on ethical issues. Or you can give them a realistic clinical scenario to role-play as a context for learning communication skills.

Do the group activities enable students to be active learners? As we discussed in Chapter 1, learners need opportunities to engage in actual learning tasks (e.g., wrestle with complex concepts, solve problems, rehearse new ways of interacting with patients). If they are to get the most out of such experiences, they need to reflect on them, assess their performance, and get feedback from others.

Determining or clarifying resources needed for the session

A variety of resources can help bring internal group experiences to life. For example, a mocked-up patient chart or a set of radiological images can help provide a sense of reality as learners work through a patient care problem. Role plays can be brought even more to life with the participation of stan-

---

[4] We recommend that learners begin having at least some exposure to the world in which they will be working as professionals as soon as possible (ideally, beginning the first weeks of school), so that all of their learning can be linked to this real-world context.

[5] Kurt Lewin (1948) was a leader in demonstrating how experiences created in groups could stimulate learning.

Table 2.1   (Sample/Partial) Plan for Small Group Discussion Session

Start time	*Activity*	*Resources needed*
9:00AM	Introductions	Name tags
9:10	Orientation	Class handout
9:20	Discussion of Topic 1, beginning with video trigger tape to establish a context	Video trigger, Monitor Videocassette player

dardized patients (Chapter 7). Video equipment enables you to review recordings of learners interacting with patients in real patient settings. Also, the group can make and review videotapes of role playing done in the meeting. Standard equipment for most small groups is a large chalkboard or a flipchart (a large pad of paper on a stand).

To ensure that you or others have thought of all the resources required, make a list of all the planned activities and the resources needed for each. For example, you can create a session plan, such as the partial example provided in Table 2.1.

Determining or clarifying the schedule for the session

As you make or review the session schedule or plan, consider the following:

Has sufficient time been allowed for key activities?
When groups meet for the first time, key components typically include:

- introductory activities (introductions, overview, orientation, discussions about how to work together)
- one or more learning activities (e.g., role plays, case presentations), including time for reflecting on and processing each activity
- summary activities (opportunities for learners to reflect on how they've worked together and what they've learned, identify learning goals that emerged during the session, and plan the next session).

When insufficient time is allowed for introductory activities, there is a risk that learners will not know what to do or will not feel ownership of the goals and strategies of the session. Also, as we discuss in Chapter 4, the first part of the session is an important time for gathering diagnostic information about learners that can guide you in refining your plans for the session so they are appropriate for the learners. For example, if you discover that learners are less knowledgeable about the topic than you had anticipated, you might decide to begin at a more elementary level and move the session along at a slower pace.

It is common to underestimate the amount of time learning activities will take, leaving insufficient time toward the end for reflecting on the activities. Without reflection, learners can be deprived of the opportunity to get the most out of an activity. Also, commonly, groups fail to preserve time for summary activities. Without adequate reflection and summaries, there can also be negative side effects, as discussed in Chapter 4.

Subsequent sessions should begin with opportunities for learners to "check in"—to review relevant experiences they've had or work they've done between sessions, report any further reflections they've had about the last session, and anticipate what's coming. Subsequent sessions should close with "check outs"—time for summary activities.

Have allowances been made for changes of pace and breaks?
Although learners' attention spans are longer when they are actively engaged than when they are passive, there are still limits to their attention for any activity. Varying the kinds of activities in which learners engage can help sustain their attention. For example, if the initial activity is serious and takes great concentration, you might choose to next have a lighter, less demanding activity. If the session is more than an hour long, be sure to include a break roughly every hour.

Is the schedule sufficiently detailed?
If the group needs to cover a lot of ground under time constraints, the session will probably need to be well structured, with a fairly detailed schedule that includes start times for each activity. On the other hand, if the session will be fairly open-ended and the group will not be under pressure to accomplish specific tasks within a fixed period (e.g., a relaxed discussion), the session can be relatively unstructured and a detailed schedule will probably not be needed.

Does the schedule allow for slippage and changes of direction?
Nonauthoritarian small groups seldom go exactly as planned. Schedule slippage can be allowed for by slightly overestimating the time allotted for activities, identifying which activities are expendable, and deciding which can be done more quickly, if necessary. Particularly if you

don't know the learners and are not sure that the session plan will be appropriate for their interests and skill levels, have optional activities available.

Determining or clarifying the focus of your leadership

Robert Bales (1950), a pioneer in studying group functioning, described groups as having two dimensions, which we refer to as the "task" and the "interpersonal" dimensions. The task embraces *what* the group is trying to accomplish; the interpersonal embraces *how* the group members communicate and interact while pursuing their tasks. All groups have both components. For example, in a primarily task-oriented group, such as one in which students are learning how to examine eyes, attention still needs to be given to how the students work together. In a more process-oriented group, such as one in which students are learning communication skills, one of the explicit tasks might be for learners to focus on how they are interacting with each other in the group. Teachers in process-oriented groups tend to recognize that they will need "people skills" but may forget the need for some task orientation. Conversely, some leaders of task-oriented groups (particularly those emphasizing cognitive content or motor tasks) do not always realize that people skills are needed for having a successful group. In subsequent chapters we deal with both the people ("process") skills (e.g., how to help students listen actively to each other) and with the task (organizational) skills (e.g., how to help learners jointly solve a clinical problem) needed by all leaders.

Determining the kind of leadership you need to provide

In Chapter 1, we discussed how educators using an authoritarian approach have one main way of providing leadership—being directive. On the other hand, the degree to which collaborative educators provide direction depends on many factors, such as the purposes of the group, the learners' levels of competence and confidence in being able to carry out the group's learning tasks, their competence and confidence in assuming group process responsibilities, where the group is in its development, and the available time. In other words, the amount and kind of direction that collaborative teachers provide is situationally determined (Blanchard, 1995). In addition, collaborative teachers serve as facilitators, helping learners develop their capacity to do things for themselves. As you reflect on the kind of leadership that you want to bring to any group you are or will be leading, consider the following questions.

When, how much, and what kind of direction to provide?

The amount and type of direction needed by learners varies with the circumstances. In general, they are most likely to need direction (modeling, demonstrations, suggestions, advice) when doing tasks for the first time or when making substantial changes in their accustomed ways of doing things. Put another way, learners tend to need direction when their competence and confidence are or feel low. There are also times, of course, when there are educational benefits to be derived from having the learners struggle with figuring things out for themselves. In effective educational planning the decision about the learners' degrees of independence and the amount of direction provided by the teacher are worked out collaboratively, guided by the intent of maximizing the benefit to the learners.

Direction is seldom needed only once. Learners are particularly likely to need direction multiple times if they are newly learning complex capabilities or if they are trying to make a major change in the way they already do something.

The kinds of direction provided by collaborative educators generally differs from that provided by authoritarian teachers. Collaborative educators seek to help learners become self-reliant as soon as possible. Toward that end collaborative educators may keep their directions brief, use language that is familiar to the learners, and frequently invite the learners' questions. They might ask learners to repeat the directions in their own words to confirm their comprehension. Collaborative educators get learners practicing what they are learning as soon as possible. Then their observations of the learners' practice provide diagnostic information that guides whatever additional coaching they offer. Authoritarian teachers, on the other hand, convey the message that they are, and intend to remain, in charge. They are likely to follow their preformed plan. Any demonstrations they offer tend to be extended and uninterrupted. They are not as likely as collaborative educators to invite the learners' self-critique of whatever practice they do, and any feedback they offer on that practice tends to be judgmental.

When to be facilitative?

We recommend facilitation as a primary and regular instructional posture. As we've indicated, even as you model a new skill or give directions, your focus can be on how to help students most quickly learn to do the skill themselves or provide their own direction. Facilitation is achieved primarily with questions that encourage learners to do their own thinking. Facilitation is also achieved by supporting learners when they take risks and try new ways of functioning or try to alter established patterns. Facilitation includes giving encouragement, praise, and constructive feedback frequently. The amount of active facilitation that is needed is likely to be highest when learners are newly acquiring, or modifying, capabilities. (This is also when they might need most direction.) As learners develop competence and confidence, they can assume more responsibility for facilitating their own and each others' learning.

Collaborative instructors are likely to be less facilitative and more directive when there are time constraints. For example, the leader might provide more direction if the group has a specific task that must be done quickly or if learners are struggling to do something themselves but time is running out. (We recommend structuring sessions so that learners have as much time as possible for the repeated practice they need for lasting learning.)

As clinicians do with patients, collaborative instructors are likely to be more directive or even take over if a potentially harmful situation arises that they think the learners are unable to handle. For example, if one group member is being hurtful to another and the group doesn't appear ready to deal with the situation, the leader might step in and be directive.

Educators can also function one way in relation to the learning tasks but another way in relation to group process tasks. For example, if group members are learning a new technical skill but have begun working effectively with each other, the leader might offer to demonstrate the new skill but ask the learners to decide how to set up the session and how to use him (the teacher) as a resource.

Determining or clarifying your tasks and roles

Throughout this book we describe a variety of tasks that need to be carried out before, during, and after group sessions. Most of these tasks typically fall to the group leader, particularly when the group first starts to meet. However, as we've mentioned, some preparatory tasks might be handled by course coordinators, other faculty members, administrators, or students. Leadership tasks during and after group sessions can be shared with a faculty coleader (see Chapter 5) or with learners in the group. Confirming in advance who will do which tasks helps ensure that the tasks are carried out and that duplication of effort is minimized or eliminated. Knowing in advance what you are to do before, during, and after group sessions can enable you to decide whether you have the capabilities needed for carrying out the tasks and help you plan your time.

The tasks you are to do are closely linked to the role(s) you will play. As we discussed in Chapter 1, key roles for educators include diagnostician, role model, and coach. When helping learners, educators go through cycles of assessing, modeling, coaching, and fading (Figure 1.1), depending on the amount of direction and support learners need. Blanchard (1995) describes four leadership roles that shift with the group's changing needs: (1) directing; (2) coaching; (3) supporting; and (4) delegating. Other roles that change with the situation are: resource person, evaluator, meeting planner, mediator, and advocate for a person or idea.

Determining or clarifying the learners' roles and responsibilities

If you and the learners are to plan and monitor their participation in the group, you and they need to be clear about their roles and responsibilities. In educational groups, the student's main role is to be a learner. Other roles (many of which support this role) include those listed previously for the instructor. In other words, learners can serve as role models and resource persons, for each other and even sometimes for the leader. Learners are likely to have many tasks related to their roles as learners and as facilitators of each others' learning. In addition, some of the leadership tasks described in this book can also be assumed by learners. For example, they can help ensure that everyone has an opportunity to participate, monitor the group's progress in completing a task, and guide the planning of the next session. Be aware of ways that learners' roles and responsibilities can change and increase over time. Also, consider ways that the learners can be involved in deciding what their roles and responsibilities should be.

Determining or clarifying how decisions will be made in the group

Although some decisions are made in advance for learning groups by faculty members, most collaborative learning groups have decisions they need to make. Even if the group's central task (e.g., discussing an article) does not require decisions, groups still need to make decisions about how they will work together. Patricia Williams (1995), an organizational consultant and physician, describes five types of group decision making:

1. chaotic (by chance)
2. theocratic (by ritual, e.g., "It's always been done this way.")

3. autocratic (by fiat)
4. democratic (by majority vote)
5. consensus (by collective opinion).

In conventional education, most decisions are made autocratically or theocratically by the teacher and program administrators. In many groups, members make decisions in chaotic or democratic ways. In a few groups, decisions are made by consensus. In some groups, members make decisions by informal consensus without being aware they are doing so. Whether someone else has already decided how decisions are to be made in your group, or you will make that decision, or you will ask the learners how they want to make decisions, consider some of the potential advantages and risks of the five optional approaches to decisions.

When decisions are made chaotically, members do not carefully think through issues, express opinions, or make reasoned decisions, creating a high risk that a poor decision will be made. Theocratic and autocratic decision making rob learners of opportunities for developing their capacities as decision makers and often result in later questioning or conflict. When done well, decision making by majority rule includes opportunities for everyone to express their opinions and can sometimes, but not always, be quicker than making decisions by consensus. However, there can be negatives to decision making by majority rule. Competition and disunity can be fostered by setting up situations in which people take sides and tensions develop as subgroups try to persuade others why their idea is best. After the decision is made, there is a risk that the dissident minority will not feel ownership of or commitment to the decision and may even work to undermine it.

Consensus decision making is a cooperative, collective attempt to arrive at the best possible decision for all involved, rather than a competitive struggle to persuade others of the correctness of one's view. The goal is *win-win* rather than *win-lose*. Group members jointly focus on the challenge or opportunity in question rather than squaring off against each other. In consensus decision making everyone's thoughts are considered important, so care is taken that every member has an opportunity to speak and be heard. Williams (1995) suggests the following steps:

1. Clarify the problem (or challenge or opportunity) ("The challenge we are working on is. . . ").
2. Gather data ("These are the factors that need to be considered. . .").
3. Establish outcome criteria ("Any good solution must. . .")

4. Brainstorm alternatives ("These are possible steps we could take. . .").
5. Evaluate alternatives ("Which steps best fit our criteria?").
6. Select ("All things considered, our best options at this time are. . .").

When working on some straightforward, simple decisions, the process can be greatly abbreviated. Step 3, for example, might be skipped altogether. Also, groups that practice consensus decision making tend to become more efficient with this process over time.

As a proposal is crafted, rather than voting for or against it, members express their level of support for it. In small groups, members can take turns briefly expressing their levels of support verbally. In larger groups, learners might put their thumbs up if they agree with the current proposal, put their thumbs sideways if they have some concerns but can live with it, and put their thumbs down if they do not agree with it and feel they must stand in the way of acceptance. Until full agreement is reached, a conscientious effort is made to learn from those who don't support the proposal and make modifications that are maximally pleasing to everyone. Those who do not fully agree with a proposal, but don't feel strongly enough to want to block it, may choose to stand aside and let it pass, perhaps asking that their views be noted or that they not be actively involved in implementation. If groups cannot reach agreement, they may decide to continue discussing the issue, gather more information, or agree to make the decision some other way.

Decision making by consensus can be time consuming, particularly with inexperienced groups, and a dissident minority can have considerable power, keeping the group from moving forward for long periods or completely. However, the advantages can be worth the investment and risk. Consensus decision making can enrich group thinking and can help build group cohesiveness and a spirit of collaboration, with an enhanced likelihood of subsequent follow-through on the implementation of decisions.[6] In addition, many decisions made by groups of health professionals in real clinical settings are best when done by consensus. So learning to achieve consensus as students can help prepare learners for making decisions in this way when later working on health teams or with others.

When deciding on the way(s) members will make decisions, there are several issues to consider: the amount of time available, the nature of the

---

[6] One characteristic of successful work teams is that most decisions are arrived at by informal consensus (McGregor, 1960).

group's tasks, the importance and consequences of the decision to be made, whether the instructional goals include helping the learners gain skills in decision making or in the consensus process, the possible positive and negative consequences of making decisions in the ways discussed, and the likelihood that consensus is achievable. If the group decides to make some or all decisions by majority rule, part of your task may need to be to minimize the possibility that the most outspoken, articulate, and/or influential (not necessarily the best informed or most thoughtful) learners may exert undue control over the decision-making process.

Determining/clarifying if and how the learners will be evaluated

If learners' work in the group will not be recognized academically, they may not give the group activities much of their attention. They may even skip some of the sessions. For example, if a course includes lectures and small groups but learners are only evaluated on the work covered in the lecture, learners might conclude (perhaps correctly) that the faculty do not regard the group work as valuable. Consequently, particularly at exam time, learners may not prepare for or attend some group sessions so they can study "what's really important" in preparation for their exams. There are exceptions. If learners are committed to a group and feel the experience is valuable, they will likely prepare for and attend most or all sessions. Also learners are likely to be more engaged and candid in support groups if they know that what they say or do will not affect their grades or promotion. In general, however, if you want learners to value their small group experiences, you and your colleagues need to recognize and reward these experiences in ways that are consistent with the pattern established at your institution. If in your program, as we recommend, formal tests and grades are not emphasized (Jason & Westberg, 1979), then the small group teaching efforts will not be at a competitive disadvantage.

If the learners in your group will be evaluated, consider the following questions.

What, if any, is your role in evaluating the learners?   Group leaders are often expected to provide learners with both *formative* and *summative* evaluation. Formative evaluation is the feedback that teachers provide to learners (such as during group sessions) to guide their learning.

(In subsequent chapters, we suggest ways to provide such feedback constructively.) Summative evaluation is the end-of-the-experience judgment you make about the quality of each learner's overall performance. If you are to provide summative evaluation that will contribute to the learners' grades and progress, they may initially and understandably be reticent about being open with you. In Chapter 4, we expand on this issue and recommend being fully candid with learners about your role.

If you are to fill out evaluation forms on learners (whether for formative or summative evaluation purposes) consider these questions:

- Is it clear what capabilities and/or behaviors you are to evaluate?
- Are these capabilities consistent with the stated learning goals?
- Are all the important capabilities and/or behaviors reflected on the form?
- Will you be able to provide the information requested on the form (e.g., will you have opportunities to directly observe learners using the capabilities you are expected to evaluate)?

If your response to any of these questions is "no," the evaluation form and perhaps even the overall evaluation approach may need to be reviewed and possibly revised.

What responsibilities, if any, will learners have for evaluating their own work? Since one of the most important capabilities needed by professionals is the ability to critique their own work in balanced, constructive ways, learners should have many opportunities to practice doing self-assessments in settings such as small groups where they can get feedback on the aptness of these self-critiques.

What responsibilities, if any, will learners have for evaluating each other's work? Under the right circumstances, learners can provide each other with helpful, constructive feedback. If learners are to do this, consider the following:

- What is being done to ensure that an atmosphere is created in which learners are comfortable providing feedback to each other?
- Have the learners previously had experience providing feedback to each other in constructive ways?
- If learners lack experience and skills in providing constructive feedback to each other, what steps can/will be taken to help them develop these needed skills?

- If learners are using evaluation forms for peer feedback, do the forms address capabilities and/or behaviors that are appropriate and that peers are in a position to evaluate?

Depending on the responses to these questions, additional planning work may be needed.

What mechanism is in place for giving learners the information collected on evaluation forms in a timely way? If learners are to benefit from the written feedback provided by others, they need to receive it promptly, while the original events on which the feedback is based are still clearly recalled.

Making arrangements for the meeting room(s)

Many schools in the health professions have a shortage of rooms suitable and available for small group teaching, so it is important to arrange for rooms as far in advance as possible. If you are involved in selecting your meeting room, try to ensure that

- the room is large enough to hold all group members and any needed equipment and other resources comfortably
- there is adequate room for the planned activities (e.g., role playing)
- needed furniture is available (e.g., chairs that are sufficiently but not excessively comfortable, a table for resource materials, surfaces for learners to write on)
- the area is quiet, and there are minimal or no distractions (e.g., windows through which learners can see distracting activities)
- the temperature in the room can be adjusted for comfort
- the lighting is adequate for the planned activities
- there is a chalkboard if needed and space to hang sheets of paper if the group will be using a flipchart for recording ideas
- there are no large, immovable pieces of furniture (e.g., a boardroom table) that could prevent you from arranging the room in the way you want
- there are power sources and extension cords for use and proper placement of any needed electrical equipment (e.g., overhead projector, video playback unit).

The physical arrangement of the room can support or oppose your intended ways of interacting with your learners. If the chairs are arranged in traditional classroom style, with you facing rows of learners, the message is clear: this will be a teacher-dominated session. When learners are looking at the backs of their peers' heads, their verbal and nonverbal communication with each other is thwarted. You are the only person the learners can comfortably see, so the flow of the conversation is likely to be directed toward you. If, however, the chairs are placed in a circle, or semi-circle, the message is: everyone will be participating. When group members have visual contact with each other—as they have in a circle—peer-to-peer communication is facilitated.

As you think through the room plan, reflect on how the group needs to work and how the arrangement of the resources, furniture, and other items in the room can best serve these purposes. If, for example, you will be using flipcharts, chalkboards, an overhead projector, or other visual aids, the circle will need to be incomplete (one-half to three-fourths) so that all members can easily see the material presented. If group members need to have books and writing materials in front of them, consider arranging the chairs around one or more tables, or arrange for chairs with integrated writing arms.

Think through where you will need to sit to best carry out your tasks and convey appropriate messages. If you plan to direct the group activities and use audiovisual equipment, you will probably need to be at the front of the room where you can do those tasks and be seen and heard easily by all members of the group. If you need to observe the group members, but won't be actively directing events, you will need to sit within the circle but not necessarily at the front of the room. If you want learners to take major responsibility for some or all of the activities of the group, you might convey that message by pulling your chair out of the circle. You might also want to sit in different places at different sessions, depending on your role in each group's intended activity.

Determining/clarifying approaches to evaluating your teaching

Just as learners need regular, timely feedback to monitor and adjust their efforts, so do you as a group leader need timely, constructive feedback on your teaching to ensure that you are being maximally helpful. Some questions to explore are

- What kinds of data, if any, will be collected about your teaching?
- What are the sources of the data (e.g., members of the group, coleader)?

- When are the data gathered and under what circumstances?
- How and when will the data be fed back to you?
- Who besides you will see this information?
- How will others use this information?
- Will anyone be available to help you review and interpret these data?

If students or others will use evaluation forms for evaluating your teaching, try to review these forms before serving as a group leader so you are aware of the areas of focus of the evaluation. When reviewing or designing evaluation forms, consider the following:

- Is it clear what capabilities and behaviors students or others are to evaluate?
- Are capabilities and behaviors that you care about addressed?
- Is it likely that the information gathered from these forms will be helpful to you in your teaching?
- Are those who will complete the forms equipped to make the judgments requested?

Arranging for (or learning about) faculty development and other support for small group leaders

When several faculty members will serve as group leaders for a course, clinical learning experience, or other instructional program, their effectiveness is likely to be enhanced if they meet prior to the group sessions to do such things as

- plan the group sessions or hear about and discuss what others have planned
- work out the logistics for the group sessions
- outline and discuss the tasks that leaders need to pursue before, during, and after the group sessions
- work on the skills needed for conducting the group sessions (e.g., through discussion and role playing).

A number of schools that use problem-based small group learning prepare faculty for their roles as tutors by having them role-play a tutorial session using one of the cases that they will subsequently use in their own teaching.

If there are multiple group sessions, group leaders can meet periodically, preferably soon after each session, while their experiences are fresh.

Leaders can talk both about what's working well and what difficulties they are experiencing. And they can trade suggestions. Such meetings can improve the overall quality of the course. Collectively, leaders can often detect problems and find solutions earlier than individuals can.

If you are coordinating a course that uses multiple group leaders, you might want to organize these kinds of activities. If you are one of the group leaders in such a course, you can request such activities. If you aren't working with others, you can seek out a seminar or workshop on small group leadership at your institution or at a national educational meeting. (For more on this subject, see Chapter 3.)

SUMMARY

To ensure that small group sessions are worthwhile and not mis-educative, and to help prevent problems from occurring, we recommend attending to a number of tasks, as summarized in the self-checklist in Appendix 2.1. Many of the tasks presented in this chapter, and listed in the checklist, involve making decisions. The vital first step is recognizing that these decisions are needed. Often, the need for these decisions goes unrecognized, so they are made by accident, by default, or too late. Of course, decisions made by default, or with insufficient care, are unlikely to provide outcomes that are as desirable as decisions that are made in advance, as a result of careful thought. Appendix 2.1 summarizes the key planning decisions that are typically needed for small group teaching.

Appendix 2.1
General Preparatory Tasks

✔ **Have I determined or clarified...**

❑ the planned group's size and mix of characteristics?

❑ who the learners are (e.g., their interests, strengths, and learning needs)?

❑ where the group experience fits into the overall curriculum?

❑ what the overall purpose is and what the learning goals are?

❑ whether the learning goals are sufficiently specific, clear, worthy, realistic, and achievable?

❑ the group learning activities (and whether they are done within a meaningful context that enables students to learn in active ways)?

❑ what resources are needed for the session?

❑ the schedule for the session (including whether sufficient time has been provided for key activities)?

❑ the focus of the leadership I need to provide (an appropriate balance between the learning tasks and the interpersonal process)?

❑ the kind of leadership to provide (how directive and facilitative to be, and when)?

❑ my task(s) and role(s) before, during and after the session?

❑ the learners' roles and tasks/responsibilities?

❑ how decisions will be made in the group?

❑ if and how the learners will be evaluated?

❑ the arrangements for the meeting room(s)?

❑ the approaches for evaluating my teaching and providing me with helpful feedback?

❑ whether there is faculty development and support for small group leaders?

CHAPTER 3

Preparing Yourself for Leading Groups

Our teaching reflects not only what we know and what we can do but who we are, how we present ourselves to others. Our personalities, proclivities, prejudices, and preoccupations can profoundly influence the process and effectiveness of groups that we lead.

Being experts in a discipline and effective in other types of instruction, such as lecturing, does not automatically prepare us for or make us good at leading groups. In fact, many lecturers have difficulty being small group teachers, often because they can't resist lecturing, even to only six or eight learners (Jason, 1962, 1964; Jason & Westberg, 1982). Being an effective clinical teacher/supervisor can help prepare us for some but not all of the tasks and challenges of small group teaching.

Becoming an effective small group teacher can take considerable effort, but the outcomes can be sufficiently rewarding to justify the investment. Effective small group leaders tend to have certain characteristics, many of which can be cultivated. Although some content expertise is often desirable, even mandatory, it alone is typically insufficient. Interpersonal process skills (i.e., skills needed for facilitating productive group interactions) are usually vital.

In this chapter we provide opportunities for reflecting on who you are and what you bring to your roles as teacher and group leader, and we discuss some specific steps you can take to enhance your effectiveness.

REFLECTING ON WHO YOU ARE AND WHAT YOU BRING

In many ways we have been implying that being an educator is a substantial challenge, demanding a high level of preparation and competence.

Teaching is likely to be done best by people who take this challenge seriously. We hope you agree. Regrettably, many of our colleagues apparently do not. They have had little or no formal preparation for their work as teachers, do not keep up with the literature on education in the health professions, and don't attend conferences on new developments in health professions education (Jason & Westberg, 1982)—behaviors that they and their colleagues would not likely tolerate among members of their primary disciplines.

Beyond having explicit preparation for being an educator and staying current with developments, we all need to bring to our teaching an eagerness to continue growing as educators. At the center of this process is a willingness to be critically reflective about who we are and what we do. We invite you to reflect carefully on the questions that follow.

Reflecting on your experiences as a learner

How we were treated as learners during our professional education can affect how we in turn treat our learners (Jason & Westberg, 1982). For example, if our dominant experiences were in an authoritarian model, we may have a tendency to replicate that model. On the other hand if we were regularly invited to be partners in teaching and learning, we are more likely to treat students in those collaborative ways. Whether or not you had opportunities to be a member of teacher-led small groups during your professional education, consider asking yourself the questions that follow.

To what extent did my teachers (group leaders):

- create a context and provide the challenges and guidance that encouraged us to take initiative in pursuing our learning, rather than only lecturing at us?
- create an atmosphere of trust in which we felt able to be open and honest with them and each other about our learning needs?
- foster collaboration rather than competition among us?
- urge and help us take as much responsibility as possible for planning and monitoring our learning?
- give us the message that we could and should contribute to each other's learning and assist us in doing this, when needed?
- encourage us to assess our own work and our group's work before offering us their feedback (which they then did constructively)?

Try to remember both the negative and positive experiences and role models you had, how they made you feel at the time, and how they may have influenced the way you now teach. Also, if you have been exposed to some teaching outside your professional area (in sports, music, computers, or whatever), reflect on these questions in relation to those experiences. As you do so, consider what your own learning preferences were (are) in those settings and compare them with what you experienced in your professional education. Many teachers tell us that in their personal learning pursuits they would not accept being treated in the ways that they were often treated during their professional education.

Reflecting on your experiences as a teacher

The way we currently teach is likely the best predictor of how we will teach in the future, unless we are determined to—and take steps to—change what we do. If you are currently teaching or have taught, reflect on your approach to and style of teaching, especially as a leader of small groups.

To what extent do I:[1]

- create a context and provide the challenges and guidance that encourage learners to take initiative in pursuing their learning, rather than only lecturing at them?
- create an atmosphere of trust in which learners feel able to be open and honest with me and each other about their learning needs?
- foster collaboration—rather than competition—among learners?
- urge and help learners to take as much responsibility as possible for planning and monitoring their learning?
- give learners the message that they can—and should—contribute to each other's learning—and assist them in doing this, when needed?
- encourage learners to assess their own work and the group's work before offering them feedback in constructive ways?

If you teach both in a health professions setting and outside this setting (e.g., as a sports coach or as a teacher in a religious program), compare

---

[1] If you find yourself concluding that the questions in this section are either incomprehensible or seem irrelevant to the teaching you do or want to do, we urge you to be patient. Perhaps some further elaboration will help clarify the centrality of these intellectual and personal issues to effective teaching. If you are thinking that many faculty manage to teach without ever being concerned about such issues, you are right. In most of our institutions faculty members are free to do a wide variety of things that all get to be called teaching. Our focus in this book is on what it takes to ensure that learners have positive, worthy, lasting learning experiences as a result of what teachers do, not on the range of activities that faculty members can get away with in the name of teaching.

how you teach in the different settings. If there are some differences, reflect on which way of teaching feels most natural and comfortable to you and is most satisfying.

Reflecting on characteristics of effective small group educators

The educator Kenneth Eble (1988, p. 6) noted:

> The great teacher, even the consistently effective one, may have a combination of personal qualities and behaviors that seem to defy analysis. If one does not demand that analysis identify the good teacher's precise molecular weight, however, one can find a firm set of attributes, intentions, principles which underlie diverse practices.

There are no recipes for and no single template for the ideal small group educator, but we propose that the following are characteristics that most capable small group educators share, at least to some extent. As you prepare for small group teaching, consider reflecting on the extent to which you have and are open to trying to enhance these characteristics.

Your enthusiasm for teaching?   Enthusiasm for teaching has been correlated with teaching effectiveness in numerous studies (e.g., Hildebrand et al., 1971; Stritter, Hain, & Grimes, 1975; Chickerella & Lutz, 1981). Effective teachers are not only enthusiastic about their subject matter but also about the processes of learning and teaching (Irby, 1978). They enjoy teaching, and they show it in many ways; for example, by bringing energy and dynamism to their interactions with students and by being generous in the time and support they give to their students.

Some questions to consider if you feel less than enthusiastic about teaching:

- Do you feel capable of enjoying teaching but are so pressured by other obligations that you can't give your teaching the time and energy it requires?
- Do you enjoy teaching but dislike the conditions under which you must teach?
- Do you feel burned out by the traditional teaching you are expected to offer but open to a different (perhaps, more collaborative) approach?

If your response to any of these questions is "yes," we urge you to do what you can, perhaps bolstered by some of the arguments presented in this book, to modify the expectations and educational climate at your institution or at least in your division.

Your caring about learners as people? The primary focus of teaching must be people, not the content of a discipline or anything else. Effective educators care about learners as people and are able to convey these feelings. They enjoy nurturing others and watching them grow. Nel Noddings (1984, p. 176) argued that an ethic of caring must guide teaching: "When a teacher asks a question in class and a student responds, she receives not just the 'response' but the student. What he says matters. . . regardless of whether it is right or wrong, and she probes gently for clarification, interpretation, contribution." In contrast, a lack of caring and respect for learners can impair learning and destroy groups. Stephen Brookfield put it this way (1986, pp. 12–13):

> A fundamental feature of effective facilitation is to make participants feel that they are valued as separate, unique individuals deserving of respect. To behave in a manner disrespectful to others, to denigrate their contributions, or to embarrass them publicly through extended attention to their apparent failings are behaviors that are, in educational terms, disastrous.

We are certainly not implying that *what* we teach or our expertise in our professional areas are unimportant. We are asserting, however, that *how* we conduct ourselves and teach are also vital. Without these components, no amount of subject expertise will be sufficient to have a positive impact on our students' learning, and we may well have a negative effect.

Your capacity for putting yourself in the learners' shoes? Psychologist Carl Rogers (1969, p. 111) said that significant learning is most likely to occur "when the teacher has the ability to understand the student's reactions from the inside, has a sensitive awareness of the way the process of education and learning seems to the student." Effective teachers know that the process of learning is unique for every student and work to understand how it is for each of them so as to be able to customize their learning experiences (one of many good arguments against large group, anonymous "teaching").

Your trust of the group? Effective small group educators respect the intelligence and experience of their students and convey the expectation that their students are able and willing to take charge of their learning. Rogers (1969, p. 164) contended: "If the leader's own philosophy is one of trust in the group and in the individuals who compose the group, then this point of view will be communicated in many subtle ways." If such trust is not communicated, the group is likely to behave defensively and their learning can be stultified.

Your comfort with empowering learners?   As we've described, in many collaborative groups, over time leaders retreat into the background and coach from the sidelines, so to speak. How comfortable are you doing that?

Your commitment to your own learning?   Effective educators are themselves lifelong learners, always actively pursuing their own learning. They are open to, even eager for, fresh ideas and new approaches. They visibly demonstrate their joy in being exposed to fresh perspectives that emerge in a group. Given that a major goal of professional education is helping learners become lifelong, self-directed learners, you can be a valuable role model for students, especially if you regularly exhibit these qualities during the small group sessions that you lead.

Your level of flexibility, adaptability, and inventiveness?
Group sessions can be unpredictable, "messy" events. Effective educators adapt to, even welcome, the surprises of small group teaching. They can make the moment-to-moment decisions needed for continuously reshaping the instructional experience to be maximally helpful to all the students. Educational psychologist Nathaniel Gage (1984, p. 88) explained:

> Teaching is an instrumental or practical art, not a fine art aimed at creating beauty for its own sake. As an instrumental art, teaching is something that departs from recipes, formulas, or algorithms. It requires improvisation; spontaneity; the handling of hosts of considerations of form, style, pace, rhythm, and appropriateness. . . .

Elliot Eisner (1985, p. 177) described teaching this way:

> It can be wooden, mechanical, mindless, and wholly unimaginative. But when it is sensitive, intelligent, and creative—those qualities that confer upon it the status of an art—it should, in my view, not be regarded. . .as an expression of unfathomable talent or luck but as an example of humans exercising the highest levels of their intelligence.

Reflecting on needed understandings and capabilities

Leaders of all kinds of groups need expertise, both in areas related to helping groups accomplish their tasks and in managing interpersonal process issues. Leaders of instructional small groups also need other skills. Consider reflecting on the following understandings and capabilities in relation to the small group teaching you have done, are doing, or will be doing.

Your ability to facilitate the completion of group learning tasks? To help groups work through and complete learning tasks (e.g., solve clinical problems, do and review role plays), you need some organizational and managerial skills. You need to be able to help groups become clear about their task(s), decide on ways of working together, maintain a schedule, resist intriguing but diversionary new topics, monitor the group's progress, and more. (We address additional task-management skills shortly.)

Your interpersonal and communication skills? Groups are social enterprises. To work well together, group members need to trust each other, communicate clearly and unambiguously, listen actively to each other, accept and even value individual differences, support each other, build together, and resolve conflicts constructively. To help groups work together in these ways, you need effective interpersonal skills. King and Gerwig (1981) reported that when they began putting more emphasis on group teaching in their institution, the faculty decided that to be maximally helpful to their students they needed to work on their own communication skills. The faculty found that developing advanced communication skills is an "ever-deepening, perpetual learning process."

Inevitably, a major way leaders help learners work well together is by helping them develop and enhance their communication skills. Thus, regardless of whether or not the learning of communication skills is an explicit learning goal of a group, effective leaders often teach communication skills, indirectly, or even directly. Such skills, of course, are vital for nearly all careers available in the health professions.

Your understanding of the world of health care and the challenges facing learners? To be maximally effective, we need to understand the requirements and joys of the world for which our learners are preparing themselves. This understanding enables us to help learners focus on key issues and to link what's happening in the group to the real world. Leaders who are not clinicians (e.g., anatomists, physiologists, ethicists, sociologists) can have important contributions to offer, but if they are not well acquainted with the context in which their information and perspectives will be used by learners, their effectiveness may be greatly reduced. Certainly, being a clinician does not guarantee that a leader understands the world facing their learners. For example, subspecialist clinicians trained traditionally (with little or no contact with primary care) may not understand the needs of their many learners who will work on the front lines of health care. Practitioners in disciplines or specialties different from the ones their learners intend to pursue may also not understand the particular challenges their learners will face.

Your ability to facilitate the learning process in small groups? Effective small group teachers of both genders fit Kahlil Gibran's (1967) description of the wise teacher: "If he is indeed wise, he does not bid you enter the house of his wisdom, but rather leads you to the threshold of your own mind." Robert Segal (1979) also speaks to the importance of facilitating learning:

> A good discussion leader does not directly convey what he knows but instead uses what he knows to convey to students what they themselves already know or can know. Lecturing, by contrast, aims unabashedly at imparting knowledge. Far from beckoning students to what they do know or can know, a lecturer tells them what they on their own presumably do not, and even cannot know.

Although he wrote the following more than 100 years ago and was speaking of one-on-one learning, the words of Joseph Payne (1883), first Professor of the Science and Art of Education at the College of Preceptors in London are contemporary and apply to group teaching and learning:

> If we observe the process which we call instruction, we see two parties conjointly engaged—the learner and the teacher. The object of both is the same, but their relations to the work to be done are different . . .[The] essential part, the appropriation and assimilation of knowledge by the mind, can be performed by no one but the learner. . . [from which]. . .it follow that he is in fact his own teacher, and. . .that learning is self-teaching. . .The teacher's part then in the process of instruction is that of a guide, director, or superintendent of operations by which the pupil teaches himself.

Ayers (1986, p. 50) compares teaching to assisting at a birth:

> Good teachers, like good midwives, empower. Good teachers find ways to activate students, for they know that learning requires active engagement between the subject and 'object matter.' Learning requires discovery and invention. Good teachers know when to hang back and be silent, when to watch and wonder at what is taking place all around them. They can push and pull when necessary—just like midwives—but they know that they are not always called upon to perform. Sometimes the performance is and must be elsewhere, sometimes the teacher can feel privileged just to be present at the drama happening nearby.

To facilitate learning in small groups, you need to understand the basic principles of learning and teaching as well as the different ways in which people learn. You need to be able to diagnose students' learning needs, design and facilitate effective learning experiences, and monitor learners' development. In addition, you need to be able to help students learn together—to jointly build knowledge, to serve as teachers of each other.

Your ability to function as a participant-observer? To guide and facilitate group interaction, you need information from two perspectives: the perspective of a group member and the perspective of an observer. You need to be inside a group so you can fully understand and appreciate what is being said and experienced. Yet, to have the information required for deciding when you might need to intervene to help the group, you must also have a view from the outside. You must be able to step back from the process and view yourself and the group with some objectivity. To be in these two roles requires a delicate juggling act. It is particularly challenging to be both the insightful, empathic observer that you must be, while also being an active leader. Playing this double role takes practice. As you may have already discovered, once you become aware of the importance of doing this double task and begin practicing, the process becomes progressively easier.

Your content (subject matter) expertise? Leading instructional small groups generally requires some expertise in the subject matter that is the focus of the session. For example, facilitating an effective discussion of an ethical issue usually requires both some knowledge of ethical issues in general and of the specific situation at hand. Certain kinds of small group teaching (e.g., teaching learners how to elicit information from depressed patients) requires not only knowledge in given areas (depression, interviewing skills), but also expertise in putting the knowledge into practice (e.g., being able to use interviewing skills to elicit information from depressed patients).

Content experts who also have the understandings and capabilities previously described can identify the knowledge and skills students need to develop, as well as the experiences (both inside and outside the group) needed for developing them. Using questions and other strategies, they can help learners explore the subject matter as well as other issues that emerge. When appropriate, they can guide students to journal articles, books, video programs, and other written and mediated resources and provide information that is not otherwise available. Content expertise is also needed for monitoring the process and outcomes. Like a good coach, a group leader needs enough command of whatever the learners are working on to recognize when and where they most need help.

Content experts, however, who don't understand the importance of being a guide and resource rather than a purveyor of information, can be tempted to give answers rather than help learners find their own answers. They also can be easily seduced into presenting minilectures on their favorite topics, denying the learners the needed opportunity to do their own exploring. In a word, content experts can be at risk of interfering with learning.

For some teachers and some kinds of small group teaching, a less than expert level of knowledge of a subject area can be acceptable, even appropriate. Howard Barrows (1988), a pioneer in the use of problem-based learning in the health professions, says the ideal circumstance is for the tutor to be an expert both in content and process. However, if that isn't possible, the next best tutor is the teacher who has good facilitation skills but is not an expert in the discipline being learned. Discussing their study of problem-based learning (PBL) at Harvard Medical School, Marc Silver and LuAnn Wilkerson (1991) noted that some of the best teachers were generalists rather than subspecialists. They postulated that generalists were perhaps in a better position than subspecialists to relate to students' needs, particularly the needs of beginning students. In comparing group discussions of subjects in which the tutors described themselves as experts with those in which they did not, the authors found that the tutors with content expertise tended to take a more directive role in tutorials. They spoke more often and for longer periods, provided more direct answers to the students' questions, and suggested more of the topics for discussion. Tutor-to-student exchanges predominated, with less student-to-student discussion.

Nonexperts may be less tempted than experts to drop "pearls," and nonexperts can perhaps more easily join students as colearners in the quest for knowledge. However, experts who are able to put themselves in their students' shoes, who can remember what it was like being a beginner, who understand the importance of and can be successful at restraining their inclinations to display their expertise, and who have the capabilities that will be described shortly can perhaps be the most effective leaders.

Your ability to serve as a role model?   Students frequently learn more from what we do than from what we say. We can shape student learning in powerful ways by modeling the attitudes and skills needed by learners. This

includes modeling effective ways of functioning in a group learning setting, modeling the intellectual and clinical skills that learners need to
develop, and, as we discussed, modeling a commitment to learning.

In tutorial groups at the University of New Mexico, tutors are
expected to serve as role models for students in such areas as "quantity and
quality of work, critical thinking, tutorial democracy, and enthusiasm and
growth" (Lucero, Jackson, & Galey, 1985, p. 53). Barrows (1988, p. 4) also
discusses role modeling in problem-based groups:

> To facilitate student independence and foster students' critical thinking and self-
> directed, continued learning, the tutor should guide his students at the metacognitive
> [think about thinking] level. The oral statements and challenges he makes should be
> those he would make to himself when deliberating over such a problem or situation
> as the one his students are working with. His questions will give them an awareness
> of what questions they should be asking themselves as they tackle the problem and
> an appreciation of what they will need to learn. In this way he does not give them
> information or indicate whether they are right or wrong in their thinking.

Barrows concludes by recommending that tutors continue offering
these challenges until their learners develop the habit of challenging themselves and each other with similar questions.

TAKING STEPS TO ENHANCE YOUR TEACHING EFFECTIVENESS

Taking some personal steps

Become familiar with the learners' world of health care.
If you think that you may not be adequately familiar with the health care
world your learners are currently working in or are preparing for, consider
reading about it, observing it, talking with others about it, or even joining it
temporarily. Some basic science teachers have even worked in the clinical
settings that their students were preparing to enter (e.g., Saffran, 1971).

Put yourself in your learners' shoes. Effective teachers are able
to see the world as their students see it. If you haven't recently done so, try
getting this perspective by putting yourself back in time to when you were
at a similar place in your career development. Of course, none of your

students will be exactly like you were, but recapturing some of your experiences as a learner—your learning history—can be genuinely helpful. What were some of the questions you and your peers were raising? What were some of your concerns? What were your hopes? What was difficult to grasp? What facilitated your learning? What blocked it? As we discussed in Chapter 1, many experts are unconsciously competent in their areas of expertise. If you think that you may be at that stage, work at backtracking to an earlier stage when you were consciously competent. Try recapturing the steps and issues you needed to be mindful of when you first learned the skills or concepts that are likely to be addressed in your group sessions.

Identify your small group leadership strengths and areas you need to address.   Previously we described how leaders need expertise both in content areas and in process skills. Some of us tend to gravitate toward and feel more comfortable with clear-cut content and tasks. Others of us are more at home with process issues (e.g., communication and relationship issues). With 15 years of experience examining 1,600 different groups, Fiedler(1981) reports that he can separate "task-motivated leaders" from "relationship-motivated leaders." Although all leaders are motivated toward both task and process concerns to some extent, he found that one of the two areas tends to be a primary motivation. Not surprisingly, he found that in highly structured situations (e.g., basketball teams) task-motivated leaders seemed to perform best, whereas, in moderately unstructured situations, relationship-motivated leaders seemed to perform best.

The Myers-Briggs Type Indicator (Hirsh, 1991), which has been used widely in the health professions, contributes to our understanding of personal preferences for ways of thinking and relating and how these preferences influence our leadership styles. The authors built their inventory on the work of the psychoanalyst, Carl Jung, who postulated that an individual's apparently random behavior is not random at all. If carefully observed, a pattern emerges that reflects each person's preferences for their sources of motivation (energy), their ways of assimilating information, their ways of making decisions, and their approach to living. Using labels to which the authors have assigned meanings that differ somewhat from our usual usage, their self-report instrument helps users identify their preferences in four domains.

Extraversion / Introversion. According to Myers-Briggs, people who fall toward the Extraversion [2] end of this continuum (called Es) tend to be energized by interacting with things and people in the world outside of themselves. People who prefer Introversion (Is) tend to be energized by their own inner world of reflection, thoughts, and ideas. Both Es and Is can serve successfully as small group teachers. However, Es typically are more comfortable with the informal conversations at the beginning of sessions, and they are more likely to draw energy from the learners' participation. On the other hand, Is tend to be effective listeners and may be more comfortable with the silence of learners quietly reflecting.

Sensing / Intuition. When perceiving or taking in information, Ss (people whose preferences tend toward the Sensing end of this continuum) rely on their five senses. They know and trust tangible, demonstrable data. Ns (those toward the Intuition end of this continuum) prefer using their "sixth sense," "intuition," or "gut feelings" when taking in patterns and considering possibilities. Both types of leaders use their senses and intuition, but each prefers and relies more on one modality than the other. Leaders who prefer Sensing are more able to focus on details and keep the group based in reality. Leaders who prefer Intuition tend to be more comfortable with open discussions, and they are often more able to present the big picture. They enjoy talking about possibilities and exploring visions of the future. They welcome discussions of philosophical, theoretical, abstract issues, while Ss typically do not.

Thinking / Feeling. People have preferences regarding how they come to conclusions or judgments. Leaders who prefer the Thinking mode of functioning (Ts) tend to decide things impersonally, based on logical analysis and principles. They place a premium on objectivity and fairness. Leaders who prefer the Feeling mode (Fs) tend to make decisions and judgments based on subjective values and circumstances and the impact that a decision will have on people. They place a premium on harmony.

Perceiving / Judging. People differ on whether they prefer taking in information (Perceiving) or making decisions (Judging). People who prefer Perceiving (Ps) tend to be spontaneous, curious, flexible, and adaptable. As group leaders they feel confined by structure. They prefer free-flowing conversation and exploration and may have trouble bringing closure to topics and tasks. People who prefer Judging (Js) tend to plan carefully, be decisive, self-regimented, purposeful, and exacting. As group leaders they

---

[2] This is the way this word is spelled in the Myers-Briggs literature.

welcome structure and are comfortable keeping sessions on task. They seek closure. They may be uncomfortable with free-flowing explorations.

In Myers-Briggs language, all of us operate in all eight areas, but we typically incline toward one end of each continuum and, to varying degrees, have developed one side more than the other. For all of us, when we choose to or need to operate from our less preferred side, extra effort is usually required. For example, when leading a highly structured, task-oriented group, leaders who are high on the Thinking and Judging ends of those continua will be in their element, while leaders who are high on the Feeling and Perceiving ends of those continua will need to work harder at sticking to the schedule and helping members stay focused on their task(s). Conversely, in an unstructured support group, leaders who are high in Feeling and Perceiving will tend to feel comfortable, but leaders who are high in Thinking and Judging are likely to feel frustrated, even irritated.

Being aware of our preferences, of the fact that there will be a range of preferences and related learning styles among the group members and that our preferences may or may not fit what is required from moment to moment while leading a small group, can help us be more adaptable, effective group leaders. This self-knowledge can also help us avoid misreading learners. For example, an instructor who strongly prefers Extraversion may misread a student who is a strong I, deciding, perhaps incorrectly, that his being quiet indicates that he's not interested in the group activity, not realizing this student's way of being engaged involves being quietly reflective about the material.

Developing your small group leadership skills. In some institutions there are faculty development workshops, consultations, or other experiences available to help you with whatever expertise you want to enhance in seeking to be a more effective group leader. Whether or not such opportunities are readily available, you can take the following steps:

1. *Identify your learning needs.* Make a list of the information and skills you want to develop and prioritize them. Be ready to modify the list as you gain added insight into your capabilities and the demands of small group teaching.

2. *Read, listen to audiotapes, and view videotapes in relevant areas* (e.g., group leadership, group dynamics, education in the health professions). See the references in this book for some ideas.

3. *Identify and work with a mentor.* Find a faculty member who is an effective group facilitator. Arrange to observe him or her leading small

group sessions and discuss your observations afterwards. Try arranging to colead a group with him or her and to get feedback afterwards on your efforts. If possible, when you feel ready, invite your mentor to witness you leading a group (live or on videotape) and help you critique the process.

4. *Engage in peer coaching* (Hekelman et al., 1994). Particularly once you have developed some basic capabilities, consider pairing up with one or more colleagues and take turns observing each other leading a group (live or via videotape), facilitating each other's self-critique, and offering feedback and suggestions.[3]

5. *Consult with an educational specialist or faculty developer.* Many schools and residencies have resource persons to whom you can turn for help.

6. *Attend a regional or national educational meeting.* There are a considerable number of educationally oriented meetings in each of the health professions. Most include workshops and seminars on various aspects of instruction, often including small group leadership.

Making other preparations for small group sessions

Review activities, resources, and materials. If you have been asked to direct activities or use resources that are new to you, you might want to seek out a faculty development session that can introduce you to these activities and resources. If no such session is available, you can seek out others to help you with specific tasks you face (e.g., an audiovisual specialist could teach you to use video equipment you need). And you can get some help in other ways, as described previously. In preparing yourself for the session you might also need to do some reading (e.g., of the articles the learners have been asked to read). Or you might need to attend lectures or other events, if they are the basis for your small group discussions.

Develop/refine the plan for the first session. Typically, small group leaders are given a general plan for the group sessions and are asked to work out the timing and details themselves, or they have to work out the whole plan themselves. If you have to develop some or all of the plan, review pages 34–40 in Chapter 2. Also, read Chapter 4 and other chapters relevant to your group session so you can anticipate what you need.

---

[3] This process has parallels to the process we suggest your learners engage in as they jointly review their patient care experiences (see Chapter 9).

Reflect on how you want to introduce and present yourself. Intentionally or otherwise, many health professions educators keep a considerable physical and psychological distance between themselves and their learners, especially when they plant themselves behind lecterns in lecture halls, often hiding most of their body. Even in clinical settings, many health professions educators maintain some degree of formality and distance, particularly in the presence of patients. Small groups can offer opportunities for more informality and intimacy with students. In fact, in some institutions, students expect such closeness with their teachers. Wilkerson (1991) reported that when some faculty at Harvard Medical School began serving as small group teachers they were taken aback by the expected informality (e.g., students calling them by their first names).

Allowing learners to experience you as a person as well as a professional can encourage them to explore their own humanity as they become professionals and can reduce their sense of emotional isolation. In hundreds of interviews with medical students and residents, Robert Coombs (1978, 1990) found that most felt they were the only ones who had feelings of inadequacy and felt under duress. This sense of emotional isolation was reinforced by their impression that their classmates appeared to be calm and self-assured. When interviewing practicing physicians about death and dying, Coombs learned that not a single one could recall hearing an instructor reveal his or her feelings about an emotionally poignant situation. They also couldn't remember being asked by a teacher to talk about their own feelings.

Some kinds of groups are more conducive to personal openness than others. In support groups, for example, the central task can include helping members talk about their personal concerns. That goal is most likely to be achieved in any group by facilitators who are willing to be somewhat revealing themselves. When deciding how open to be, remember that a desirable goal is helping groups be learner-centered rather than teacher-centered. Leaders who keep bringing the group's attention back to themselves can delay achievement of that goal and the positive effects that can follow. This discussion is not meant to imply that you should feel under pressure to reveal truly private information. You are simply encouraged to be as candid as you feel comfortable being in sharing events and reflections that confirm your humanness, that help learners experience you as an authentic person, and that provide them with a model of a professional who recognizes that there is more to health care than facts and figures. If you do so, you will likely be rewarded with genuine gratitude and trust, which can form the launch pad for meaningful, lasting learning.

Learn the learners' names. Calling learners by their names helps in building relationships with them. If you do not know the learners, review their list of names in advance. Even consider making or having the learners make name tags with a thick pen and large letters that can be read from across the room. If you are comfortable doing so, and it is not too contrary to your program's culture, invite them to use your first name. In some situations, this can help facilitate fuller communication.

Anticipate developments that might occur. Run through the session in your mind. Try to anticipate any problems that may arise and ways that you might prevent or handle these problems. Consider rehearsing what you might say or do.

Prepare yourself and the room immediately before the group session. Many of us have multiple, demanding responsibilities. To ensure that you are fully present with the learners and not distracted by your other pressures, arrive early if possible. Take a few minutes to clear your head and focus on your plans for the upcoming session. If privacy won't be available when you arrive at the meeting room, try going through this preparatory process in your office or on your way to the meeting room.

As discussed in Chapter 2, the physical arrangement of the room can support or oppose your intended style of interaction with your learners and deserves your attention. Even if you asked others to prepare the furniture and equipment in the meeting room, allow time in case the arrangements are not as you requested. (Also consider asking learners to help rearrange the room, as needed, as a contribution to their ownership of the process.) If you are using a video playback unit, an overhead projector, or other equipment, arriving early gives you a chance to check that everything is there, working, and ready to use.

SUMMARY

Our effectiveness as small group leaders depends on several factors: our leadership skills, our knowledge and understandings in the areas being discussed, our level of psychological sophistication, our communication skills and style, our attention to the details of room and resource arrangements, and more. In the self-checklist in Appendix 3.1 we summarize many of the steps you can take in preparing yourself to be an effective small group leader.

Appendix 3.1
Preparing Yourself for Leading Groups

✔   ## Have I...

☐   reflected on my own experiences as a learner, particularly in educational small groups?

☐   reflected on my own experiences as a teacher?

☐   reflected on the characteristics of effective small group teachers?

☐   • my enthusiasm for teaching?

☐   • my caring about learners as people?

☐   • my capacity for putting myself in the learners' shoes?

☐   • my capacity for trusting the group?

☐   • my comfort with empowering learners?

☐   • my commitment to my own learning?

☐   • my flexibility, adaptability, and inventiveness?

☐   reflected on the understandings and capabilities I need?

☐   • my ability to facilitate the completion of group learning tasks?

☐   • my interpersonal and communication skills?

☐   • my understanding of the world of health care and the challenges facing learners?

☐   • my ability to facilitate learning in small groups?

☐   • my ability to function as a participant-observer?

☐   • my content (subject matter) expertise?

☐   • my ability to serve as a role model?

☐   put myself in my learners' shoes and worked at becoming "consciously competent"?

☐   identified my small group leadership strengths and areas still needing to be addressed?

☐   worked at developing/refining my small group leadership skills?

☐   reviewed the activities, resources, and materials needed for the sessions?

☐   developed/refined the plan for the first session?

☐   reflected on how I want to introduce and present myself?

☐   learned the learners' names?

☐   anticipated developments that might occur?

☐   prepared myself and the meeting room immediately before the session?

CHAPTER 4

Leadership Tasks, Challenges, and Strategies During Group Sessions

Before meeting with a group for the first time, some leaders report the following kinds of concerns:

- What if I can't get group members to talk and participate?
- What if a few learners dominate the session?
- What if some learners don't talk at all?
- What if the group discussion or other activity goes off track?

Some instructors who are comfortable giving lectures admit that they are uneasy about having to lead groups. When leading groups they worry that they will not have sufficient control.

Group sessions are complex human events, so like life itself they can present surprises and be messy, and sometimes chaotic. Even with skillful leadership—actually, especially with skilled leadership—groups seldom proceed neatly in lecture style from one topic to another, which some teachers can find uncomfortable.[1] Although fostering learning in small groups can be demanding, it is not an impossible challenge. In fact, as teachers begin to understand group dynamics and develop leadership capabilities, they typically find that facilitating groups can be stimulating and rewarding.

---

[1] Of course, all spontaneity and surprises can be removed from groups by authoritarian leaders who maintain strong control. Except, then you don't have a group experience, you have something like a didactic lecture, but made even less efficient by the small group size, and "mis-educative" by seeming to confirm that the learners are meant to remain passive.

In this chapter we attempt to bring order to the seeming chaos of group leadership by providing a systematic way of thinking about groups and group leadership. Our approach is to identify and discuss basic leadership tasks as well as strategies for accomplishing these tasks. (In subsequent chapters we revisit some of these tasks in the context of groups that have specific areas of focus, such as problem-based learning, communication skills teaching.) Attending to basic leadership tasks, such as building trust and fostering collaboration, can help reduce or avoid many potential difficulties. We also deal specifically with the task of diagnosing and managing behavior that affects the group process negatively.[2]

The amount of time and energy you spend on the various tasks and the strategies you use are likely to be affected by the amount of time you have, the major purpose(s) of the group (e.g., discussion, support, problem solving), the learners' prior experiences with groups and with the topics being addressed, the extent to which the group is primarily task- or process-oriented, the extent to which the group is to be structured or unstructured, and your experience and skill in leading groups. For example, if you will only have a single, 1-hour session and your group task is clear cut, you probably won't want to spend much time orienting learners or developing strategies for working together.

Here, for brevity, we discuss most tasks as if they were the teacher's responsibility. However, it is appropriate and desirable to help learners become skilled in and acquire a sense of responsibility for doing most of these tasks themselves.

Building trusting relationships and fostering collaboration

As we discussed in Chapter 1, meaningful learning usually involves risk-taking. (As Mark Twain observed, you can not learn ice skating—or most anything else important—without stumbling many times in the early stages.) Learners are most likely to take the risks involved in serious learning—in trying departures from their accustomed patterns — if they understand that significant learning involves risk-taking and if they feel that you and their peers will support them through their initial awkward phases. Learners are least likely to take risks if they feel they may be put down or ridiculed.[3]

---

[2]See also Tiberius (1989) for a discussion of dealing with problems that arise in groups.
[3]Much of the inadequacy and hurtfulness of authoritarian teaching comes from those teachers who make learners feel badly for performing intellectual or clinical tasks suboptimally, even during their early stages of learning new ways of functioning. Not surprisingly, many learners work at hiding from such teachers.

If you are teaching in a highly competitive, noncollaborative environment, creating trust between yourself and your learners and among the learners may be difficult. Learners are likely to test you repeatedly (e.g., take a small risk and see what you do) before they relax and trust you. If learners act in hurtful ways toward each other, you may need to intervene, particularly during the initial sessions. Later, learners who have come to value the trusting climate may intervene themselves whenever that climate is disrupted. Many of the tasks addressed in this chapter can help to build trust.

In Chapter 1 we also introduced the importance of collaboration and presented some of the characteristics of collaborative small groups and contrasted them with authoritarian groups. In Chapter 2 we noted that being a collaborative leader requires us to adapt to the learners, not the other way around. Particularly if learners are not accustomed to being active learners in groups or are new to the topics and tasks being addressed in the group, we might initially need to be fairly directive.

We have already discussed some ways of fostering collaboration (e.g., arranging the furniture so that you are not in a position of authority and so that learners can easily see each other). Later in this chapter we talk about involving learners in formulating goals, developing ground rules, monitoring the group's progress, planning the subsequent sessions, and other leadership tasks. Following are some additional ideas.

Listen carefully and respectfully to learners.   Collaborative leaders convey the sense that all members of the group are valued individuals who can contribute to each other's learning. Such leaders take obvious delight in learning from their students, and they sincerely consider all the opinions expressed, even those they disagree with (e.g., "That's contrary to my understanding, but I want to think about it.").

Help learners recognize when they are being collaborative.
If learners are not accustomed to working collaboratively, they may need help recognizing what it is and when it is occurring. Whenever learners build on each other's thinking, help each other think through a complex issue, or jointly solve a tough problem, you can invite them to reflect on what has just happened or point it out to them.

Help learners become increasingly more responsible for the group.   To some extent, good teaching involves working toward becoming unnecessary. Ultimately, our learners need to be equipped for functioning independently of their teachers. Learning to do so is a gradual, sequential process that needs to begin as early as possible in their professional education. In small groups, learners need to become more responsible for the products of the group's efforts as well as the ways the group functions. We can help them do this by gradually increasing their leadership responsibilities and encouraging them to do more teaching of themselves and each other. This does not at all mean abdicating our responsibilities; it does mean gradually exerting less direct influence as the learners become ready for and accept more responsibility.

Beginning the first meeting with a new group

The opening moments of a group session, like the opening moments of a patient encounter, can be critical; they can set the tone for the rest of your time together. We get only one chance to make a first impression, and some first impressions are hard to overcome. For groups to get off to a good start, learners must feel welcome and be clear about why they are meeting, what they will be doing, how they will be working together, and what kind of facilitator you are. If you and the group members do not know each other, introductions should be one of the opening events.

Welcome learners and providing an overview. A warm, friendly greeting when learners first arrive can help put them at ease. It can be the first step in earning their trust. A brief, clear overview of the major goals of the session(s) can help them understand and begin developing ownership of the purposes of the group. But be brief. Avoid overwhelming the learners. A long introduction can suggest that this will be a traditional, teacher-centered (boring) class. If you genuinely feel and convey your excitement about the experience you will be having together, your energy will likely help capture their attention.

Introduce/present yourself. The step of introducing or presenting yourself can begin with giving your name and perhaps your title or affiliation. It is also an opportunity to reveal some other brief information about yourself (e.g., how your work, interests, and background link with the focus of the sessions) to set the tone for how you would like to work together and to model how you would like learners to introduce or present themselves. Carl Rogers (1969, p. 106) recommends not hiding behind a professional mask but being an authentic person with your learners, "not a faceless embodiment of a curricular requirement, not a sterile tube through which knowledge is passed from one generation to the next."

Some issues to consider when deciding what to say and how to say it:

- the amount of time you have as a group (the briefer the time the briefer the introduction)
- the kind of relationship you want to establish/maintain with the learners (e.g., how personal or collaborative you want the relationship to be—see Chapter 3)
- the "tone" you want for the meetings (e.g., will this be a formal or relaxed environment? Is humor acceptable/welcome?)
- the type of leadership you want to provide (e.g., controlling or democratic).

Invite learners to introduce/present themselves.   Even if you and the learners know each other somewhat, brief self-introductions by everyone can help break barriers to participation by giving everybody some initial air time, establishing the premise that everyone has something to offer and is invited to be an active contributor. Once people have spoken, they usually find it easier to speak again. Introductions are opportunities to begin getting to know learners as people and to gather diagnostic information. For example, you can ask learners to tell what they enjoy doing outside of school, and/or you can ask them to briefly talk about their experiences with the topics or skills being addressed in the group. Also, to see if they have expectations for the session(s) or goals for themselves, you can ask them what they hope to get out of the session(s). Introductions can be a time to begin focusing on the session's topic. For example, in a group on communication skills, you could ask learners to break into pairs, spend 2 or 3 minutes interviewing each other, and then each introduce to the group the person they interviewed.

If you do not know the learners and they are not wearing easily readable name tags, when they introduce themselves you can list their names on a seating chart. (Referring regularly to this chart can help you learn their names.) Also, as the learners talk about themselves, you can make shorthand notes about their expectations, special interests, concerns, and other information you want to remember.

Discuss how the learners will be evaluated.   In some programs this is the learners' area of greatest concern and is best dealt with early. If learners will be evaluated, give them a summary of the competencies and behaviors that will be the focus of the evaluation, the criteria that will be used, who will evaluate them, and how they will be evaluated. Show them any evaluation forms that will be used. Early in the session it's usually sufficient to discuss the overall scheme and answer their pressing questions. You can present additional details later.

Determining learners' experiences, needs, strengths, and interests

Being diagnostic is one of our central tasks as teachers. The more we know about our learners, the more we are able to customize the group experiences to their needs. Even if you gathered information about the learners prior to the first session, there is probably more that you need to know. The following are some issues and strategies to consider.

Listen to and observe learners prior to the start of sessions.
The way learners carry themselves (e.g., comfortably, tentatively) can provide clues about who they are and what they need. Their informal, pre-class conversations can help alert you to their concerns about the group as well as external issues that might intrude on the session. If, for example, they have just taken a difficult exam, they might need to process that experience before they will be ready to participate fully in the work of the group.

Gather information at the opening of the first session. As we suggested, you can gather some diagnostic information during introductions. You can also pose diagnostic questions to the whole group. Learners are likely to be most forthcoming and to give you what you need if they understand why you are asking these questions. Before gathering this information, consider saying something like, "I want our sessions to be on target with what you need and what you are interested in. I can best help do that if you could briefly summarize what experiences you have already had with . . . ."

Use information you gather. Learners are most likely to be fully candid if they believe that what they tell you will be used constructively. For example, if learners tell you that they have had negative experiences in prior groups, you might immediately explore ways to help ensure that your time together will be as positive and productive as possible. *Caution*: If learners have had negative experiences in your institution, try to structure the conversation(s) in ways that will avoid personal attacks on others.

Begin all sessions by being diagnostic. Even when beginning subsequent sessions, be diagnostic. Although you can gather some helpful information by observing learners before sessions begin, for additional information consider beginning sessions with a "check-in"—asking learners how they are doing, whether there have been any important new developments since your last meeting, whether they have had any reflections about the last session that they want the group to know about. Such check-ins help ensure that you are aware of any feelings, issues, or events that might have a direct or indirect impact on the session. (Some leaders refer to this task as "taking the group's temperature" or "getting their vital signs.")

Maintain a diagnostic posture.   Throughout all sessions, try including careful attention to the ways the learners participate as well as what they say and do. Your ongoing diagnostic attentiveness needs to focus on a wide array of issues and events, ranging from differences in attentiveness and participation among members, to each person's communication style and intellectual patterns, to subsurface themes that reappear in the nonverbal elements of their communications. Throughout, avoid any temptation to treat hypotheses as if they were confirmed information about the learners. Hypotheses need to be tested before they are used to guide instructional actions. For example, if you suspect that some learners do not understand a particular concept, ask some questions that give you access to their thinking about that issue before taking other steps.

Helping learners understand or develop learning goals

If the learners are to pursue preformulated goals that you or others developed before the first session, your leadership tasks include helping the learners understand and feel ownership of these goals. If the learners develop their own goals, then one of your tasks is facilitating this process. In either case, you need to ensure that the group members understand and support the rationale for having goals. Some key steps in accomplishing these tasks are outlined next.

Discuss preformulated goals.   Consider distributing copies of the preformulated goals. Ensure that the learners understand the goals and the goals' relevance to their careers. (If the goals are not clearly relevant, they need to be revised.) If appropriate, help the learners feel ownership of the goals by having them think through how the goal(s) can help them be more effective in their future work. Find out if any of the learners feel that they have already, or almost, accomplished some of the goals. Goals that are too advanced or too elementary for group members should be modified.

Develop learning goals. As we discussed in Chapter 2, learners need to develop the habit of formulating their own goals. If they will be doing so in your group, you may want to

- find out what experiences they have had devising learning goals
- help them understand the rationale for setting their own goals as part of becoming lifelong, active learners if they do not already value doing so
- challenge them to think about what they want to get out of the session(s)
- give them some examples of learning goals to help them get started, if necessary.

Note: Some learners might be *unconsciously incompetent*; they may not yet have any idea what they need to learn in the area proposed for your group. They may need to have some experiences inside or outside the group that will confront them with the importance of—and their need for—the knowledge and capabilities they do not yet have, thereby helping them move to the learning readiness stage of being *consciously incompetent*. Learners are best able to formulate goals for themselves when they are aware of what they need but do not yet have. Helping learners transition into this stage can be our most important task; and it is certainly one of the most neglected, in the early stages of learning in new areas.

Discussing, deciding how to work together

In the absence of information about what is expected of them, learners can become frustrated and even take on undesirable roles. Some may, for example, revert to being "passive learners"[4] and get angry if you don't behave in traditional, authoritarian ways. To help prevent frustration and confusion among your learners, consider the following strategies.

Discuss strategies/activities for achieving learning goals.

If the learning activities you will be using were planned in advance, one of your tasks is acquainting the learners with those plans: what you and they

---

[4] We drew attention to the phrase *passive learner* since it is widely used, but it probably should not be. It is an oxymoron. Although learners may certainly behave passively, in doing so they interfere with or prevent meaningful learning.

will be doing. You may also need to help them understand the value of these activities. If they are to help plan the activities, you may need to begin by providing some guidance in how and why they are to engage in these tasks. (See "Determining or clarifying the group learning activities" beginning on page 38.)

Discuss the learners' role(s) and responsibilities.   If there are preformulated expectations for the learners' behavior, make those expectations as clear and concrete as possible. For example, if learners are expected to be active participants in the group, and they are not accustomed to learning in that way, describe in concrete terms what that means (e.g., active participants ask questions, participate in role playing, etc.). Rather than merely saying that learners are responsible for the success of sessions, indicate what that behavior looks like (e.g., if a learner thinks that the session is not going well, she speaks up and works with others to make the session more productive).

If roles and responsibilities are not preestablished, consider talking through the tasks that need to be accomplished and how best to distribute the work. Again be as specific as possible. (For maximum value, learners should take on new roles that will stretch them.)

Discuss your role(s) and responsibilities.   Talk with the learners about your role(s) and responsibilities. If you will be functioning in a way that is new to them (e.g., as a facilitator of learning rather than a purveyor of information), discuss the rationale for this way of teaching and the implications for how you will work together. If you anticipate making changes in what you do (e.g., as the group is ready, moving from being directive toward nondirective), you might also discuss how your role will evolve and why.

Discuss/develop ground rules.   Ground rules (operating agreements) are overtly stated, agreed-upon ways of working together. Some examples are

- Arrive on time.
- Listen carefully to each other.
- Try being curious (not judgmental) about others' views.
- Provide everyone with a chance to participate.
- There are no "dumb" questions.
- Don't interrupt.

- Don't monopolize the session.
- Don't discuss any private group information outside the group.
- Don't discuss any group members in their absence.

Ground rules exist to enhance the group's effectiveness, so they may need to be revisited from time to time, and the members should be encouraged to regard the rules as subject to challenge and revision if needed.

If ground rules have been developed in advance by faculty members, one of your leadership tasks is helping the learners understand these rules and become committed to following them. If any suggested ground rule is contrary to the general norms of your institution (e.g., you propose that members do not put each other down, but learners regularly belittle each other in other classes), this topic may need an extended discussion. If no rules have been developed, consider helping the group develop them. You might, for example, ask learners to reflect on the conditions that will make it easiest for them to work together productively, put those conditions into some simple statements, and then secure agreement on their willingness to adhere to these rules.

Decide how you will make decisions together. If members will be making decisions together, you and the group will need to take time to decide on the decision-making approach that will be used, or review the rationale for the approach that others have decided must be used. In Chapter 2, beginning on page 42, we discussed some of the advantages and disadvantages of decision making by majority rule and consensus. Regardless of which method is used, be sure that all learners have an equal opportunity to present their proposals and reactions, and that everyone gets a fair hearing.

Develop learning contracts. Contracts can document the group's goals, roles, responsibilities, and ground rules. Groups may have explicit contracts, implicit contracts, or both. Explicit contracts are openly stated, even put in writing. Implicit contracts are assumed to be understood and accepted by everyone but are unspoken and unwritten. Although topics such as goals, roles, and norms may never be discussed, they may eventually become sufficiently clear that members recognize when any have been violated. For example, in some groups an unspoken (and counterproductive) norm evolves prohibiting members from directly challenging each other's thinking. If members are seen to be coming to the defense of those whose thinking has been directly challenged, a leadership task is helping them recognize that this unarticulated norm exists and that it's consequences need to be thought through.

In some groups, despite the presence of an explicit contract, there is an overriding implicit contract. For example, the leader and learners might explicitly agree to share leadership tasks, but the leader continues functioning in authoritarian ways, and the learners accept (at least outwardly) their traditional, passive roles. Or the group members agree to be nonjudgmental about questions and comments introduced by group members but gradually revert to their pattern in other courses of being demeaning toward members whom they regard as too eager or conscientious.

Unless one of the purposes of the group is to see what kind of implicit contract evolves, we recommend jointly developing explicit contracts with learners. (Particularly if learners are new to working in groups and with contracts, it might take more than one session for them to understand the importance of and to develop a contract.[5]) Then, you need to be vigilant in ensuring that you and the learners adhere to the contract. If you or they have trouble living within the contract, discuss what's happening and revise the contract if you agree that it is no longer realistic or fully appropriate.

In the best of circumstances, Christensen and colleagues argue (1991, p. 21), contracts become covenants. He was talking about large discussion groups at Harvard Business School, but what he said is relevant to small groups in health professions education:

> When we let students share in the governance of their own course, they are less likely to feel like second-class citizens. And since people who contribute to setting standards often feel moved to surpass them, the best teacher-student learning contracts can also transcend themselves. When this happens, they evolve beyond formal procedures, legality, and details of enforcement to become covenants rather than mere contracts: solemn compacts among members of a group to pursue common goals for mutual benefit. Covenants promote the deep commitment that encourages accountability and mutual responsibility. They nurture true community, for who will reveal his innermost beliefs, dreams, doubts, and most adventuresome ideas in an atmosphere of distrust?

Facilitating the learners' active participation

A recurrent nightmare for some leaders is being faced with a group of silent, bored learners who can barely wait for the session to end. We have

---

[5] Developing learning contracts in groups may have the positive spin-off of helping students value and learn to develop contracts in other learning situations. Such contracts are associated with competence in lifelong learning (Fox & West, 1983; Westberg & Jason, 1993). Further, developing learning contracts might even help prepare learners for developing contracts with patients.

discussed how learners are most likely to be active if they feel safe and feel your support and the support of the group. They also are more likely to participate if they are helped to understand that participation is both expected and helpful to them and the group. Following are some strategies to consider.

Build sessions around issues that concern the learners.
You are most likely to get the learners' attention if you start with what they view as relevant and important. In later chapters we offer suggestions of several ways to accomplish this vital instructional task. In Chapter 7 we discuss building learning around patient care and other clinical problems that may have been designed by faculty, or based on real situations. In Chapters 9 and 10 we explore ways to build learning around the learners' own experiences with patients and others.

Use resources that bring issues to life.   Most learners in the health professions are preparing for careers of direct involvement with practical clinical tasks and responsibilities, not for theoretical or abstract explorations. Video trigger tapes presenting interactions with patients can help capture learners' attention and give them concrete situations on which to anchor and build discussions. Even provocative poems and excerpts from stories or plays can serve this purpose (Chapter 6). Video triggers and standardized patients can help both bring problem-based learning to life (Chapter 7) and facilitate the learning of interpersonal skills (Chapter 8). Making video recordings of learners as they interact with standardized or real patients can help learners see themselves as others see them and refine their communications skills (Chapters 8 and 9).

Use questions more than statements.   Declarative assertions from teachers, especially when used often, tend to reinforce learner passivity. Intriguing and provocative questions, on the other hand, provoke curiosity, inviting learners to participate—to share their thinking, examine their beliefs and assumptions, consider options, and ask their own questions. Questioning is usually most effective when it involves a sequence of linked questions. Educators DeTornyay and Thompson (1982, p. 77) noted:

> The impact of questioning lies not in its single acts, but in the manner in which the skilled teacher is able to combine the types of questions into a pattern. These include the particular combination of focusing, extending, and lifting from one level to another.

Foster interaction among learners. In collaborative groups, learners interact with each other, not just with the facilitator. In Chapter 6 we describe ways to encourage dialogues among learners, rather than their talking one at a time with you. In Chapter 7 we discuss how learners can use problems and cases to learn with each other. Throughout Chapters 6–10 we talk about learners sharing experiences and information, and their providing feedback to each other. Role playing is yet another effective strategy for promoting meaningful interactions among learners (Chapter 8).

Determine why some learners don't participate—or seem not to participate. As you try involving all group members in sessions, you might find that one or more learners don't participate or participate relatively little. There are many possible reasons for learner non-participation. They may be tired or bored, not understand what they are supposed to do, or they may not have prepared for the session (e.g., they did not do the required reading). Seeming nonparticipation may also be related to their cultural background, their gender, their way of receiving and processing information, or their way of relating to people. For example, a learner who is not participating verbally in a discussion might be from a background in which it is considered impolite to raise your voice or push your way into a conversation (which might be necessary in a talkative group). Other nonparticipating learners might have grown up in families in which all conflict was strictly avoided, so they stay out of lively debates (which they regard as verbal sparring). Or seeming nonparticipation may be gender related. Tannen (1990, 1994) describes how boys and girls are socialized differently, resulting in different ways of talking and being with others. This leads some women to initiate conversation less than men, to wait to be recognized before speaking, to back off when they are interrupted, and to behave in ways that might cause their contributions to be less noticed. They are also more likely to avoid conflict.[6]

Another possibility when you notice learners who participate little — and perhaps do not even look interested—is that they keep their energy and enthusiasm inside and don't always reveal it on their face. Their lack of verbal participation might be related to their preference for thinking carefully about each topic before responding. Perhaps they are listening

---

[6] For further reading on issues of diversity see Coles (1986); Takaki (1987); Nabakov (1991); Cross (1994); and Ritvo and colleagues (1995).

intently but don't yet feel that they have something to say (in Myers-Briggs terms[7] they prefer Introversion—see page 65 and Hirsh, 1991). Or if the conversation is highly theoretical, perhaps they are learners who prefer functioning in the world of the five senses, with things that they can see, hear, and touch (Ss in Myers-Briggs terms), and they are uncomfortable with theoretical or abstract issues.

The essence of this discussion has been to re-emphasize the importance of the leadership task of being diagnostic and to expand the meaning of this vital task. Whenever we experience learner behavior that is not expected or is not welcome, we need to withhold our judgments and begin gathering information that may explain that behavior. We must be willing to look beyond our learners' surface appearances and to challenge our initial hunches and hypotheses, although, of course, they may sometimes be right.[8]

Helping learners from different backgrounds and with different styles be part of the group

Being different is a relative phenomenon. Some of the learners we just described may not feel at home in a particular group or when engaging in a particular activity but would feel at home in another group or with another activity. If some learners in your group are not participating and you suspect that their non-participation might be due to differences between them and others in the group, reflect on the culture of your small group. Is it primarily exclusive or inclusive? Does it shut some learners out or make some learners feel uncomfortable? If so, what can you and the group do to open up the culture so everyone can feel welcome? Also reflect on your own background and style, and the extent to which you might be regarding some learners' behavior as problematic largely because they are different from you. For example, it's not uncommon for teachers who focus much more on people than things to regard learners who focus more on things and principles as unfeeling (and, consequently, as unappealing).

In later chapters we discuss ways to draw on and build on learners' diverse backgrounds. Here we likewise suggest drawing on and building on group members' diverse styles, finding ways to use all of their strengths. For example, again in Myers-Briggs terms, people who prefer Introversion

---

[7] We have chosen to cite the Myers-Briggs Type Indicator because it is widely used in the health professions. Also see Kolb's learning style inventory (1984).

[8] Dispensing a prescription without first doing a diagnostic evaluation is every bit as inappropriate in education as it is in clinical practice.

(Is) might say little in a group, but if group members give them a chance to talk (e.g., provide some adequate pauses) or draw them out, these learners might prove to have a good deal to contribute. Ss might tune out of some abstract discussions but they can help the group stay honest about facts and details, and as noted earlier, resources such as video triggers and case summaries can provide the concrete examples that can engage their interest in more abstract issues. Learners who enjoy change and innovation (Ns) can stimulate the group with new challenges. Learners who prefer making decisions based on the logic of the situation (Ts) can help the group think systematically about problems, while learners who are particularly sensitive to the people issues (Fs) can help facilitate the group process. Learners who are curious and adaptable (Ps) can help the group examine new possibilities. Learners who tend to be decisive and purposeful (Js) can help the group plan and monitor its progress and complete its work.[9] Helping learners recognize the value of and use each other's strengths can maximize the group's sense of inclusiveness and the effectiveness of the learning experience. Helping learners develop all of these capabilities in themselves is also likely to enable them to function more effectively on health teams.

Monitoring the flow of the session and the group process

Being a group facilitator can be demanding and preoccupying. While giving full attention to some aspects of a group, some events can be overlooked and lead to unintended, undesired outcomes. Interpersonal problems can develop among group members. Meetings can run out of time without important tasks being accomplished. Our enthusiastic involvement with some particularly verbal learners can leave others feeling neglected and discouraged. As we discussed on page 61, leaders can best monitor the group process by functioning in the dual roles of participant and observer. They can also enlist group members to help with some of the monitoring responsibilities. The following are some elements of these tasks.

Monitor the group's progress in relation to the agreed-upon agenda, schedule, and contract. Agendas, schedules, and contracts are only helpful if used. The task of watching the clock to ensure that the group is on schedule can easily be shared with learners. One or more of the learners can also help monitor the group's adherence to the terms of the contract.

---

[9]For more on the implications of the Myers-Briggs preferences for learning and teaching styles and techniques, see Lawrence (1982) and Kroeger and Thuesen (1992).

Reflect on your experiences in the group. In your role as participant, you can get some feel for what it is like to be a member of the group, particularly if you're trying to imagine yourself in the learners' shoes. Some questions to consider:

- Is the current activity holding my attention?
- Do I feel that we are making progress toward our goal(s)?
- Am I experiencing any strong feelings (e.g., anxiety, anger, boredom, restlessness) that might be a clue to surface or subsurface issues for the group?

Sometimes it is helpful to check your feelings and perceptions with the group ("I am feeling like we are getting bogged down in this discussion. Is anyone else feeling this way?").

Be aware of what you may be communicating. To help ensure that your behavior is congruent with your intentions, try remembering to reflect regularly on what you say and do, and, especially, how you say what you say. Remember, nonverbal messages are more believable than verbal messages (Beebe & Masterson, 1993). About 65% of the social meaning of messages is communicated nonverbally (Birdwhistell, 1970); and when a verbal message contradicts a nonverbal message, people are more inclined to believe the nonverbal message. For example, if you want to be collaborative, are you conveying genuine interest when you are listening or might you be showing some impatience? Are you avoiding sitting or standing in positions of authority? Is your tone of voice as inviting of learner participation as your words?

Observing the learners' behavior

The learners' verbal and nonverbal behaviors can provide important insights about the current state of the group as well as clues about the group's future directions. When you observe positive behaviors, you can encourage them. If you detect potential sources of difficulty, you may choose to take appropriate corrective or preventive action. The following are some questions to consider as you observe groups:

1. *To what extent are learners engaging in behaviors that facilitate the group process?* Some examples: eliciting ideas from others, listening attentively, rephrasing a statement to facilitate understanding, asking for clarification, volunteering to participate in constructive group activities such as role playing.

2. To what extent are learners engaging in behaviors that can have a negative impact on the group? Some examples: arriving late, leaving early, not paying attention, having private conversations, digressing from the topic or the group task, dominating discussions, cutting others off when they are trying to speak, arguing excessively.

3. Are any learners adopting consistent roles? Are any learners behaving in routine ways, such as serving as initiators (bringing up new topics); protectors (trying to protect others in the group); devil's advocates; humorists; or diverters (taking the group off its tasks)?[10]

4. How do learners relate to each other? Who do learners listen to most carefully? Are there members to whom others defer? Are there members who are ignored or whose opinions are discounted? Are any members emerging as leaders? Do you sense any sibling-type rivalry?

5. How do learners relate to you? Are any of them excessively deferential to you? Do any learners treat you like a parent? If so, what kind? Are any behaving competitively with you? Are any consistently questioning or challenging what you say?

6. What messages are learners conveying nonverbally? Group members spend more time communicating nonverbally than verbally (Beebe & Masterson, 1993), so pay close attention to their facial expressions, body postures, movements, and seating patterns. Depending on cultural and other factors, some members are likely to be more revealing than others in their body language. Observe the behavior of both those who are speaking and those who are not. Look for clues about individuals and groups by observing where learners sit in relation to you and in relation to each other. For example, learners who do not want to be or do not feel part of the group may literally move their chairs away from the other learners (e.g., outside the circle). Learners who are seeking your attention or approval may sit next to you. (They may sit there for a variety of reasons, so avoid jumping to hasty conclusions.) Subgroups (cliques) of learners might try to always sit together. When groups have developed high cohesiveness all members might put their chairs close together. Learners who are in conflict may sit far apart.

Remember when observing learners, initially we can only hypothesize about the meaning of the behaviors we observe. To understand the meaning of behaviors, we must watch for consistency over time and check with the learners (e.g., "Some of you seem puzzled. Are you?" "I'm sens-

---

[10] This is a frequently quoted classification of role types, developed by Benne and Sheats (1948).

ing some tension in the group. Anyone else feel it?"). Again, you must have achieved a high level of trust before you can expect fully candid responses to such questions.

7. *How are learners affecting each other's behavior?* Groups develop distinctive personalities and work patterns. Wheelan (1990, p. 15) observed: "At some level we understand the quality of wholeness a group embodies. We refer to groups as if they were single entities, speaking with one voice." For example, it is common to hear established groups referred to as being competitive, rebellious, quiet, and so on. H. L. Nixon (1979, pp. 4–5) noted:

> Groups have a character of their own, distinct from the personalities or qualities of their individual members. And...this 'group character' can have a significant impact on how individual members feel, think, and act, both individually and collectively.

Because groups are a type of system, systems theory offers a guide for interpreting what you observe. A group, like a system, is made up of elements or parts joined together by a relationship of interdependence. Whatever happens to one element in a system has consequences for other elements (or persons) in the system. Because of their interdependence, the behavior of each learner is linked with the behavior of all others in the group. There is no such thing as pure nonparticipation. A member sitting silently with eyes averted can have a powerful impact on other members of the group.

Systems (groups) are always striving for dynamic equilibrium or balance. When the behavior of one group member changes, the dynamic equilibrium of the group may be upset. This change can threaten the stability of the group and may be resisted by members who may engage in compensating behavior. If, for example, one member who has long been quiet becomes actively talkative, others who were dominant may become abruptly withdrawn, or even vigorously competitive, to regain their former prominence.

Reflect on the evolution of the group. Groups are dynamic organisms that grow and change. Students of group dynamics agree that "healthy" groups, particularly those that have multiple meetings, typically evolve through stages. Most groups do not go neatly from stage to stage. Groups can be in more than one stage at a time, and they can skip stages. Some groups, like individuals, can get stuck in an early developmental stage and never move on. Adding new members to a group and other changes or

Table 4.1 Stages in Group Development

Source	Stage 1	Stage 2	Stage 3	Stage 4
Fisher (1991)	Orientation	Conflict	Emergence	Reinforcement
Peck (1987)	Pseudo community	Chaos	Emptying	Real community
Thelen & Dickerman (1949)	Forming	Conflict	Harmony	Productivity
Tuckman (1965)	Forming	Storming	Norming	Performing
Wheelan (1990)	Dependency/ Inclusion	Counter-dependency/ Fight	Trust/ structures	Work

stresses can set groups back into earlier stages. Although there are multiple formulations of group stages presented by different authors (see Table 4.1), there are considerable parallels among them. Knowing something about these stages can help you interpret your learners' behaviors and facilitate the development of your groups.

Stage 1. Members are not sure what they are supposed to do. They seek direction. Most members are tentative and polite as they struggle with issues of acceptance, approval, and inclusion. They try to size up the leader and other members and determine rules, roles, goals, and structure. Typically there is initial dependence on the leader. Members may direct their comments through the leader, and they study the leader's reactions to them and the others. They seldom disagree with each other in this phase but, instead express their ideas ambiguously. It is as though they do not want to offend others or incur their disapproval by stating a definite point of view, or they do not want to take a position that they might have to repudiate later. At this stage, humor may be used to avoid intimacy and reduce intensity.

Stage 2. Members now struggle with the group's tasks and how to work together. Most researchers agree that power and control are issues here. In a task-oriented group there is conflict about the task, how it should be done, and the roles of group members. Members might compete for leadership and control. They tend to make more direct, unambiguous statements and may polarize on opposite sides of an issue. It is not uncommon for members to become angry with the leader and to display this anger directly or indirectly.

Stage 3. If conflicts are resolved, groups move to a stage of *trust* or *harmony*. Peck (1987) says members empty themselves of barriers to communication. Tuckman (1965) says members begin to develop norms and rules and become a cohesive unit (*norming*). Wheelan (1990) says they develop structure.

Stage 4. If groups move successfully through the first three stages, they reach a stage of *productivity, performing, work*. Peck says that a "soft quietness descends."

When working with new groups you can use your knowledge of these stages to guide your decisions about appropriate steps to take, such as the following. Consider beginning with trust-building activities. Encourage learners to express differing perspectives early in constructive ways. Watch out for "groupthink." You might delay some activities (e.g., asking peers to give feedback to each other) until members are no longer vying for power and trust each other. To help learners through the stages, alter your leadership style to match what the group needs. For example, as learners begin taking more responsibility for the group, consider being less directive, serving more as a coach. Then, as they become focused and in harmony, consider fading—getting out of their way. If you join a preestablished group, determine what stage the group is in. Be aware that the group dynamics are likely to change when you join them (e.g., they may begin testing you and be less trusting of each other until they are comfortable with you). Remember that group building takes time and is not a linear process.

The amount of time a group will spend in each stage, or whether they will make it through all stages, is not usually predictable. Time and progress vary with the experience and characteristics of the members, the skills of the leader, and even the total time available for the group. If group members know they have only four 2-hour sessions together, they may make it through the early stages more quickly than a group that knows it has twenty 2-hour meetings.

Facilitating the flow of the session

Observing and reflecting on the group's progress and process can provide information you need for facilitating the flow of the session. You can choose to encourage the group to be self-reflective and make its own discoveries about what is happening and what to do about it, or you can share what you observe. You can take action yourself ("Let's move on to the next topic") or wait to see if the group acts. The following are some strategies that can contribute to group progress.

Interrupt the group and ask for their reflections on the process.
Typically members get so caught up in what they are doing that they do not reflect on what's happening. To help them become more reflective and responsible for the process and any problems that might be developing, stop occasionally and ask them to reflect aloud on what is happening. This step can be particularly helpful if the group goes off track, if interpersonal conflicts develop, or if the group reaches an unrecognized decision point.

Provide feedback to the group.
Feedback can help the group reflect critically on its own functioning. Most feedback should be *descriptive;* it should provide a description of rather than a judgment about what you observe. ("Three times Maria has tried to tell us about her patient who has Alzheimer's. Each time she tried, someone changed the subject. Do you have any thoughts about what might be happening?") Leaders can also describe their internal reactions. ("When the group starts rehashing this issue, I get frustrated and worry that we won't finish on time.") Feedback can also be interpretive (i.e., leaders attribute meaning to what they see). ("The ways you're discussing the patient's problem suggests to me that you aren't comfortable dealing with the pathophysiology of this condition.") And feedback can be *evaluative* (i.e., leaders make a judgment about the behavior they observe: "I really appreciate the way that all of your presentations have included sensitive attention to the impact of the patients' condition on their families.").

When giving feedback, do so in a caring, supportive way. Avoid embarrassing learners. Focus on their behaviors, not labeling them or judging them as people. (*Use:* "Each time someone gave you feedback, you came back with a complaint about something they had done, without indicating that you were trying to learn from their comments." *Not:* "You are so defensive that you are not hearing what people are trying to tell you.") Be aware of whether your feedback is descriptive, interpretative, evaluative, or a mixture. When providing descriptive feedback, be as specific as possible. Use neutral, nonjudgmental language. When possible, after presenting descriptive feedback, invite learners to make their own interpretations or evaluations, before you offer yours. Doing so can provide you with valuable diagnostic information about their level of self-awareness and can give them practice using the vital skills of self-assessment.

When providing interpretative or evaluative feedback, link it to a description of the event or behavior so learners can better understand your thinking. Since, as we discussed, we can usually only hypothesize about the meaning of the learners' behaviors we observe, present any possible interpretations as tentative questions, not conclusions (e.g., "I wonder if some of you are uneasy about talking about Alzheimer's disease?"). Treating hypotheses as if they were facts can be risky. For example a leader who tells the group, "You are clearly uncomfortable talking about people with Alzheimer's" risks being wrong, loosing credibility, and causing learners to be defensive.

Most feedback, even so-called *objective feedback*, is subjective to some degree, it is influenced by our own experiences and filtered perceptions: what we choose to look at, what we see, and how we interpret it. Try being aware of the subjectivity of any feedback you offer and label it as such. ("It appears to me....", "I feel....", "I think....")

Keep the group focused on intended purposes. It is easy for groups to get side-tracked. You may need to remind members of their agenda. ("You have brought up an interesting topic, but we said that today we would focus only on the ethical issues related to responding to patients who want to end their lives.") If the diversion is important, you might want to find a way to deal with it later. ("That is a very important issue but we have some other things we must get done in our last half hour. Would one of you be willing to look into this new topic and report back to us at the next meeting?")

Help the group transition to new topics or tasks. Before proceeding to a new topic or task, consider stopping and summarizing what has occurred so far, or ask the group to do so. Then provide, or ask a group member to provide, an introduction and transition into the next topic or activity. One way to keep track of what has been accomplished, particularly in a task-oriented session, is having someone write down key points or issues on a chalkboard or flipchart whenever they are introduced. Then, when you want to move on, you have a record of what the group has covered.

Discuss alternative directions. When a clear branch point has been reached, if the group is not set on getting a specific task done immediately, it may be appropriate to pause and devote some group time to agenda setting. You might say, for example, "Three important areas have come up in this meeting. Clearly, we can only deal effectively with one at a time. Let's spend a few minutes deciding which one to deal with first."

Make mid-session changes in goals and/or strategies.
Sometimes the group is diverted by issues that can not wait. If the group is going off in a direction that appears to need prompt attention, call the members' attention to what is happening, or encourage members to discover what is happening. Then jointly decide what changes to make in the plans for the session to accommodate for this unexpected development.

Provide changes of pace, if needed.   If group members appear restless or tired, try finding a way to change the pace. If you are using video triggers, you can introduce a new one. Sometimes learners can be helped by a fresh infusion of energy, perhaps from a brief story or joke. If the session has been intense, long, or both, consider giving the learners a stretch break. Most people need a break, even from engrossing sessions, about once every hour.

Dealing with learners who are affecting the group process negatively

Although many problems in group leadership can be prevented by attending to the kinds of tasks described previously, problems can still occur. Here we suggest some generic steps to consider when responding to learner-related problems.[11]

Be diagnostic.   Trying to solve a problem in a group without first understanding the origins and nature of the problem is equivalent to prescribing medications for a patient without first doing an assessment. Rather than offering a quick intervention, try to figure out what is going on and what might be at the root of the problem. Just as clinicians generate hypotheses about the sources of patients' problems as part of their diagnostic workup, effective group facilitators also begin generating hypotheses about the sources and meaning of their learners' behaviors. Observing a learner who dozes off during a class and doesn't participate in the discussion, a facilitator might speculate that she is bored and uninterested, or that she is tired from being post-call, or that she has been partying too much.

---

[11] See the entries identified under "Challenges" in the index for examples of various instructional challenges.

Of course, having hypotheses is not the same as having a diagnosis. Some hypotheses can be tested indirectly. For example, if you suspect that a learner is being overtalkative because he is nervous, help put him at ease and see if he becomes less talkative.

Some hypotheses need to be tested more directly, either during or after the group session. Some learners need to be told what you observed. For example, if a learner is dozing and not participating, you might call her aside after class and say something like, "Maria, during the last two sessions you dozed off a couple of times, and you have not participated in the discussions." Sometimes this will be enough to elicit an explanation. At other times, you might need to add a more direct invitation, "Is there anything you would like to tell me?" or "What do you suppose is going on?"

If you suspect that a learner will be embarrassed by a discussion of your observations during class or has an issue that he or she would not want to share with others, it's usually best to arrange to talk privately. You might also choose private meetings with learners if a public intervention might be disruptive or insufficiently constructive for the group.

Carefully observe what is happening. When learners engage in disruptive behavior, such as monopolizing the conversation, sleeping, or talking privately (cross talking) during group discussions, be aware not only of what the learner is doing, but how his or her behavior appears to be affecting other group members, including you. Such observations are usually your first diagnostic step. The more specific and objective your observations of the learners' behaviors are, the more helpful your feedback can be.

Characterize the problem. You need specific information about the problem behavior. Is it new or long-standing? Is what the learner doing (or not doing) most likely a one-shot event or might it be repeated in the future? Are others being meaningfully affected? In what ways? How disruptive is the behavior? Does the behavior seem to be provoked by specific events or people? Your interventions, of course, will vary according to your answers to such questions.

Get to the source. Dealing effectively with problem behaviors usually requires understanding the source of the behavior. For example, learners who monopolize conversations might have a strong need to control others, or they might enjoy talking and be unaware that their enthusiastic outbursts are at other people's expense. Or they might be uneasy in the group and have a pattern of talking excessively whenever they are tense. A gentle strategy is likely to work with learners who enjoy talking or are uneasy. With them, it is often sufficient to say something like, "Thanks for getting us started. Let's now hear how the others feel about this issue." Although you might also start with a subtle approach with learners who are controlling, ultimately you might need a more direct, forceful approach (e.g., "Jim, when you talk a lot, others do not have a chance to participate").

Wait for group members to intervene.   It can be tempting to try to quickly fix problems that are occurring in your group. Sometimes this temptation is fueled by learners who pressure leaders to fix problems. For example, some learners get frustrated, even angry, with leaders who do not take care of problems that affect them negatively, such as members who are taking more than their fair share of the limited available airtime. However, if we intervene too quickly, we can rob learners of the opportunity of learning how to handle their own problems, and we can deny them the satisfaction of being successful in doing so. If possible, before intervening yourself, allow some time for the learners to recognize what is happening and make their own efforts at seeking a solution. If they do not take the initiative, you can encourage them to do so before taking explicit action yourself (e.g., "Should we be taking a look at how this session is going?").

Intervene in stages.   Interventions can range from gentle and subtle to explicit and forceful. For example, if two learners talk privately with each other from time to time during a class session, some possible, sequential interventions could include

- catching their eye (but not communicating any facial sentiments) while they are talking so they see that you are aware of what they're doing
- giving them nonverbal feedback (e.g., catching their eye again, but now frowning)
- reminding the learners about the ground rule (only one person should talk at one time), assuming that the group articulated such a ground rule
- giving them verbal descriptive feedback of what you observe (e.g., "When you talk I have trouble hearing what others are saying." ... said gently and nonjudgmentally, at least at first)

- giving them descriptive feedback of your internal reaction (e.g., "When you talk while others are talking, I get annoyed because it is quite distracting.")

Sometimes the diagnostic strategy of describing the learners' behavior to them can be sufficient, especially if they are not aware of how they are being perceived or of the impact their behavior is having on other people.

Unless the situation is out of hand, consider starting with a subtle intervention. If that does not work, raise the ante. If appropriate, allow time after each intervention for group members to intervene. Also ensure that the way you intervene is constructive and doesn't destroy the climate of trust. If learners consider your actions arbitrary or unfair, your relationship with all group members could be damaged.

Before intervening, consider the possible consequences of what you plan to do. All but the most subtle types of intervention are at risk of disrupting the group process. Reflect on such questions as: What might be the impact of interrupting the process? Is it worth it? Are there any risks that the intervention might be more hurtful than helpful?

Manage the group's shifting loyalties. One of the more complex challenges of being a group leader involves monitoring and adapting to the group's shifting loyalties. Initially, if you have not worked with them, the learners may feel loyal toward each other and perceive you as something of an outsider. During this phase, if you do anything that is interpreted as an attack on a group member, even a disruptive one, the group may turn on you, and regaining their trust may then be slow and difficult. Once you have crossed the threshold of being seen as genuinely on their side, as their advocate and as someone who can be trusted, you can then takes steps on their behalf—and may even be expected to. For example, you might help squelch a bothersome member, providing you are seen as doing so fairly and decently. Even after you have earned their trust, if you are newly discovered to have a latent potential for harshness or unfairness, you will slip back badly in their estimation, since most or all members may then see themselves as vulnerable. Skilled leaders are always alert to signs of the group's attitudes toward them and toward each other. They are careful not to exceed the group's level of trust or indulgence, but they do intervene on the group's behalf, when their help is needed.

Reinforce positive behavior. If learners who had been difficult make positive changes in their behavior, let them know that you recognize and appreciate these changes, either in private or in the group, depending on your judgment of which is more appropriate.

Dealing with disagreements and managing conflicts constructively

Each of us sees the world in a unique way, so when two or more people try working together, there may be disagreements. In instructional groups, members (including the leader) may disagree about the purposes of the session, strategies for achieving goals, the way the group should work together, the ground rules, the leadership style that should be provided and more. Members may also disagree about content issues (e.g., the accuracy of information presented by a member, the validity of a piece of research, the efficacy of various patient care interventions). As we've already suggested and will discuss further later, such disagreements can be instructive. In fact, we encourage leaders to elicit multiple points of view and to help learners listen carefully to each other.

In some situations, learners can agree to disagree. For example, in a discussion about ethics, members may disagree strongly about whether health professionals should assist patients who want to be helped to die. After listening to each other, members may simply agree that they each have valid points of view, given the assumptions and premises with which they each begin. However, there are situations when group members must come to some form of agreement before being able to proceed with their work. For example, if they are going to jointly work through a patient care problem, they have to decide how they will proceed and what each member's responsibilities will be.

Earlier we suggested that groups decide on a process for making decisions together. If this process allows for everyone's point of view to be heard, if there are ground rules about how members communicate with each other, and if the process is regarded as fair by all members, disagreements are not likely to escalate into hurtful events.

Conflicts between group members or between yourself and one or more learners are potential opportunities for growth and for helping members learn to negotiate the inevitable differences between themselves and others. If the conflict is handled well, groups can emerge more cohesive and productive, and members can learn ways to deal with conflict constructively that can carry over to their interactions with patients and peers. However, mismanaged conflict can lead to hurt feelings, emotional withdrawal from the group, reduced cohesiveness, and general disruption of the learning process.

Identify the nature of the conflict and who's involved.

Since the way conflict resolution is approached needs to be congruent with the nature of the conflict, it is important to identify the parties to the dispute, the focus of the dispute, the possible roots of the dispute, its severity, and its duration.

Typically to resolve a dispute in a satisfactory way, the key parties to the dispute need to be identified and involved in its resolution. When identifying the disputants, it's tempting to focus only on those learners who are arguing or displaying their dissatisfaction openly. Be aware that others (inside or outside the group) may be important to understanding the dispute. For example, two learners might be acting out a conflict that actually involves most or all of the group members. Or if the group is to resolve its dispute about the way learners are being evaluated, the course coordinator who designed the evaluation scheme might need to be involved.

Learners can be in conflict about goals, information, or structural issues (e.g., how to accomplish a task). They can also be in conflict about real or perceived differences in values or interests. Or conflicts can be linked to personality or relationship issues. Generally, the more that the conflict involves challenges or perceived challenges to how learners view themselves or want others to view them, the more difficult it is to deal with and resolve the conflict. For example, resolving a conflict about information (e.g., the accuracy of the information that a learner presents to the group) is usually far easier than resolving a conflict that involves differing perceptions of a learner's competence for doing a group task (e.g., gathering and summarizing information for the group).

As you try to sort out the nature of a dispute, be aware that many conflicts include more than one area (e.g., learners may be in conflict both about their goals and how they want to achieve their goals). Sometimes you can deal with one conflict area at a time; in other situations all conflicts may need to be dealt with together.

Also be aware that the area of conflict that is most apparent (e.g., a heated argument about the accuracy of certain information) might be fed by much more fundamental conflicts (differences in values). For example, two learners might be arguing about the definition of universal health care, but the root conflict might be linked to differences in their values (e.g., one learner feels a moral obligation to provide health care to everyone, the other learner feels that only those who "pay their own way" have a right to health care). To face or resolve conflicts meaningfully, the parties usually need to focus on the root or foundation of their conflicts, on their *interests*, not their *positions*. (More on this topic shortly.)

The duration and severity of the conflict should likely shape how you approach it. For example, it is usually best to deal immediately with a new, minor conflict before it escalates. And you might need to dedicate most or all of a group session to a severe, long-standing problem.

Create an environment in which learners can discuss disagreements early, before they become conflicts.   Most problems are easiest to manage in their earliest stages. In instructional groups, however, some learners avoid acknowledging and dealing with disagreements promptly out of concern that there will be negative consequences for being in conflict with the leader or other group members (e.g., their grade may be lowered or the person with whom they are in conflict may retaliate).

Building trusting relationships can help some learners feel sufficiently secure to acknowledge problems before they become formidable. In addition, as we discuss later in this chapter, taking time at the end of every session to reflect on how group members are working together can help bring issues to the surface early enough to be managed easily.

Help learners listen to each other.   A conflict can often be resolved if the parties take time to listen carefully to each other and try putting themselves in each other's shoes. This can be done informally during a group session. For example, if two contentious learners don't appear to be listening to each other, you might interrupt and say something like, "The two of you don't seem to be listening to each other. Would you be willing to take a few minutes to make a special effort to hear each other?" If the learners agree, you can structure an exercise, such as the following. Ask Party A to describe his view of the situation without Party B interrupting. Then ask Party B to repeat what she heard. And then ask Party A to indicate whether Party B heard correctly. If Party A does not feel fully or accurately heard by Party B, the process can be repeated. Then ask the parties to switch roles. Ask the parties to use "I" language and to refrain from making inferences about what the other party was thinking or feeling.

If multiple people, perhaps including you, are involved in a dispute, similar opportunities can be arranged for taking turns speaking and listening actively. Also, if there are more than two points of view, all views need to be presented. If it doesn't seem necessary or possible for the listeners to paraphrase what they've heard, they can demonstrate in other ways that they've listened actively (e.g., ask for more information, request clarification).

Conflicts are often diminished or resolved when parties feel that they've been heard by the others in the dispute. If the conflict involves relationship issues, being heard means that each party becomes aware of how the other person felt (e.g., hurt, angry). The parties often realize that they had not been communicating clearly with each other. Sometimes this involves realizing that they had not been aware of the impact of their behavior on other people. When this happens, the parties may apologize spontaneously.

Help learners negotiate a solution. If learners are in deep conflict, you might want to work with them outside of the group or refer them to someone with skills in conflict resolution. If you are in a protracted conflict with a learner or learners, you might need a third party to mediate. Fisher and Ury (1990) suggest doing the following.

Separate the people from the problem. Before working on the substantive problem (if there is one), disentangle the people (relationship) problem and deal with it separately. Then the parties can come to see themselves as working side by side in dealing with a common issue rather than facing each other down.

Focus on interests, not positions. People who are in conflict typically each take a position, which they tenaciously defend. The more they try to convince the other side(s) that it is impossible to change their opening position, the more difficult it becomes to do so. When arguing over positions in the hope of improving their chances of getting what they want, parties often start with or adopt extreme positions and then drag their feet. As in bartering in the market place, negotiating over positions involves successively taking and then giving up a sequence of positions (making concessions) to reach a compromise. Disputes that focus on positions often produce unwise or incomplete agreements, if any.

Instead, when negotiating over *interests*, each party needs to be clear about what they need or want and why these underlying interests are important. Such negotiations should begin by having the learners in the dispute educate each other about their respective interests. Help them identify common or complementary interests (e.g., that they both want to learn during the group sessions). Frame the problem in a way that can lead to a win-win solution. ("What will it take for you both to get what you want?")

Generate a variety of possibilities before deciding what to do.
The most creative part of the process can be jointly proposing ways to deal
with the conflict that will satisfy as many interests or needs as possible for
all parties. Encourage the parties to brainstorm many possibilities before
reaching an agreement. Invite them to invent options that will bring maximum mutual gain.

Follow-up with the learners who are in conflict. After the learners work out a solution, devise a way that they and you can check later to
see how they are doing.

Facilitating the achievement of the learning goals

Our major task as educators is helping learners develop the capabilities
they need for being safe, effective health professionals who remain so
throughout their careers. Accomplishing this substantial goal, and all the
subsidiary goals that are involved, in a timely, effective way can be challenging. The following are some steps involved in fulfilling learning goals
in the group setting.

Keep the goals in mind.   As we've discussed, formulating new goals
or reviewing preformulated goals at the beginning of a session can help
guide learning during the session. If as the session is underway the group
goes off track, revisiting the goals can help get learners back on track, or
lead to the decision, if appropriate, that the original formulation needs to
be revised.

***Foster self-assessment and provide constructive
feedback.***   As we've also discussed, for students to become competent
lifelong learners, they need to have the habit of routinely reflecting on and
assessing their success in achieving their learning goals. Doing self-critiques during small groups gives them practice with this vital skill and
enables them to feel the dignity of being the ones who identify any
deficiencies they have. Hearing the learners' self-critique gives us
information about their mastery of this skill, which can then be the basis
for any feedback that we or their peers offer.

In some groups self-critique and feedback are structured activities.
For example, in groups in which the learners' goals include developing
communication and interviewing skills, learners practice interviewing each
other or standardized patients. Following the interview, the student inter-
viewer assesses his interview and then receives feedback (oral and perhaps
written) from the leader, the other learners, and the standardized patient

(see Chapter 8). Also, in some groups at the end of some sessions or at the final group session, learners might do oral and written self-assessments, give feedback to each other, or both. Leaders may also provide informal or formal feedback.

In most groups, any self-critique or feedback that occurs is less systematic or formal. For example, a learner might spontaneously declare that he still doesn't understand a particular concept. In other groups self-critique and feedback don't occur at all…but should. Since learners need repeated practice in doing self-assessments and in providing feedback, we recommend including these activities routinely in learning groups.

The following are some steps in preparing learners for self-assessment and feedback:

- Ensure there is a climate of trust.
- Determine the learners' experiences, comfort with, and attitudes toward self-assessment and giving feedback to each other.
- Deal with the learners' misconceptions, hurtful prior experiences, and negative attitudes toward self-assessment and peer feedback.
- If needed, help learners understand the value of self-assessment and feedback.
- Ensure that learners understand what they are to critique.

When reviewing learners' progress with them, try routinely inviting their self-critique before offering your feedback. Encourage them to comment both on what they did well and what still needs work. When you give feedback to learners, provide a model of what you recommend as their way of giving feedback to each other. When learners are expected to give feedback to each other, explicitly talk through how to do so constructively.[12]

Processing and summarizing what occurred during the session

Too often learners leave a group session without a clear sense of what has been accomplished, either in terms of content or process. Some learners might complain that they "didn't get anything out of the session." Members often have different perspectives on sessions and take away unique impressions of what happened. In many groups, time is not protected for summarizing and reflecting on what occurred. Without that "processing" time, potentially valuable events can quickly fade from memory and be lost. The following steps can help enhance the lasting value of group sessions.

---

[12] We discuss self-assessment and feedback in more depth later in the book.

Allow sufficient time.   When there is a great deal for groups to do during a session, it can be tempting to try saving time by reducing or eliminating whatever time may have been scheduled for processing and summarizing. Time needs to be carefully protected for these activities. When learners flit quickly from one experience to another, without time for reflection, important lessons can be lost. Often there are many threads of conversation that need to be pulled together for them to make most sense and be retained. For example, in task-oriented sessions, members need to review where they stand in terms of completing their tasks or goals. In process-oriented sessions, such as support groups, it's important to determine whether any learners have unfinished business for which follow-up plans are needed. Skipping session wrap-up time can also leave learners without a sense of closure.

Make sure learners understand why time should be taken for summarizing and processing.   If the learners have not been prepared for allowing wrap-up time at the end of their sessions, they can be upset at a leader who interrupts an engrossing discussion before the session's designated ending time. Learners are less likely to be frustrated if the leader made the rationale for such wrap-up activities clear at the beginning of the session and agreement was reached on the time this activity was to begin.

Reflect with learners on what the group accomplished.   If the group had specific goals, reviewing them can help members appreciate what they've accomplished and determine what still needs to be done. If the group didn't have specific goals, members can still talk about the achievements of the session. The group's sense of accomplishment can be enhanced with a summary on a flipchart or chalkboard of what they've done.

Reflect with individual learners on what they learned.
Asking each member to briefly identify one or more key things that he or she is taking away from the session provides you with potentially helpful diagnostic information about individual learners as well as the group. Also, hearing what their peers gained can help learners consider issues they might have missed initially, and reinforce important "take-home" messages.

Reflect with learners on how they worked together.   Reflecting on the process can provide you with insights about the learners' awareness and understanding of the process and with ideas about how to improve the process at the next session. If there are ground rules, you might want to start by reviewing them (e.g., "We agreed that we would take turns talking and listening carefully to each other. How did we do?"). You might also ask learners to indicate, aloud or on paper, what factors facilitated or blocked their learning (i.e., what they, you, and their peers did that helped or hindered their learning).

Share what you've learned and reflect on how you worked together. You can underscore the collaborative nature of groups by sharing some of what you learned. You might also want to comment on how you and they are working together. For example, a leader might say, "As you know, I want you to assume increasing responsibility for the group. I realize that sometimes I jump in when you could be handling things yourselves. I'm trying to catch myself, but may need a reminder from you at times. And I encourage you to try not turning to me for answers, at least initially. Try first to work things out for yourselves."

Make plans for follow-up and the next session. If the group is going to meet again, decide what each member of the group will do between sessions. Also, if appropriate, decide what you want to deal with or accomplish at the next session and what strategies you will use to achieve these goals. Use what you learned during the summary to decide how to work best together. Ensure everyone understands when and where the next session will be. If you want subsequent sessions to start on time, negotiate a reasonable start time with the learners and then begin promptly, even if not everyone is there.

Take time for your own reflection and planning. As soon after the session as possible (while your memory is still fresh), jot down observations and thoughts that will help you plan future sessions of this group or your own functioning in future groups. Some group facilitators find they are helped by keeping a log of each session, much like clinicians keep careful records of patient encounters. Consider creating a form with space for: (a) tasks/strategies that went well; (b) tasks/strategies that didn't go well; (c) follow-up steps/tasks to take; (d) specific reminders about individual students; (e) a list of students who were absent; and (f) general notes.

Closing final group sessions

Most of the steps previously discussed also apply when conducting the final session in a series of group sessions. During a closing session, however, the group is likely to be best served if the reflections focus not only on the present session but on the group's entire time together. You can help your learners consolidate their maturation as group participants and prepare for future groups by posing questions such as the following:

- What have we accomplished during our time together?
- How would you describe the ways we worked together?
- Have there been any changes in the ways we've worked together? (Has the group gone through any changes, such as the stages in the life of a group noted earlier? Have learners assumed increasing responsibility for the group?)
- What are some of the most important lessons you're taking away from this experience?
- How do you plan to apply what you've learned?
- Do we as a group and/or you as individuals have any unfinished business?
- How can we handle that unfinished business?
- What would you want to do differently in your next learning group?

The final session should include opportunities for learners to critique their own performance, their peers' performance, and your contributions as a facilitator. This can be done both aloud in the group and on evaluation forms. There should also be opportunities for you to provide feedback to the learners, both aloud in the group and privately with each learner.

Terminating Close-Knit Groups

Long-term groups, or even short-term groups whose members have developed strong, close bonds may find it difficult to terminate their group. Some groups that were set up for specific, time-limited tasks decide they will continue meeting even after the initially agreed-upon tasks have been completed.

When groups have gone well, their endings can bring a sense of loss. Even if the learners will continue to have contact, the group identity and experience will end. Common reactions to the feelings of loss that such endings can bring are grieving and anger (e.g., "You're abandoning me.") (Sampson & Marthas, 1977).

In close-knit groups, members may deny or avoid dealing with termination. Some symptoms of denial or avoidance can be the emergence of negative behavior: lateness, apathy, refusal to engage in deep or meaning-ful discussions, and premature withdrawal. Learners who formerly talked rather openly and easily may become defensive and superficial. Members may appear to be angry, with no apparent reason. Conversations may shift toward discussions of death, dying, failure, and loss. Some learners may make plans for additional meetings of the group (Sampson & Marthas, 1977).

Sufficient time needs to be allowed for learners to deal with their feelings. An open-ended question might help get this task started ("We've been together for quite a while. What is it going to be like for you not to have this group any more?"). If members are denying or avoiding facing termination issues, you may need to confront them. ("I've noticed that people who typically were talkative aren't saying much today, and our discussion keeps shifting toward death. Do you have any ideas about what might be happening?") If the group has trouble making the connection but you sus-pect there is a link, you might say something like, "Sometimes people in a group that is preparing to end realize that they're going to miss the group. Could that be a factor here?"

Evaluating the learners' participation and capabilities

As we discussed in Chapter 2, prior to the first session you need to be clear about any evaluation tasks you are expected to perform. Items on evalua-tion forms are usually presented cryptically, so if you are expected to fill out a form that others developed, ensure that you understand any vague items (e.g., "communicates well with others"). If necessary, ask for spe-cific criteria that translate into behaviors you can observe. Strategies that can help with serving as an evaluator include taking a few notes about learner performance throughout the sessions, as long as doing so does not inhibit the learners or cause discomfort. Also, or alternatively, it is important to get into the habit of making notes about the learners' and group's experiences as soon after all sessions as possible.

SUMMARY

Many educators, especially those new to small groups, worry about the challenges they might face. Problems certainly can and do occur during small group teaching. Group sessions are complex human events, so, like life, they can offer surprises, be messy, and sometimes be chaotic. Groups seldom (and certainly shouldn't) proceed neatly in lecture style from one topic to another. Yet, most problems can be prevented with adequate planning and skilled leadership, and most problems that arise can be managed. The basic tasks involved in leading small groups effectively are summarized in Appendix 4.1, in a self-checklist.

·As is undoubtedly all too clear from a careful reading of this chapter, being an optimally effective facilitator of learning in small groups involves attention to a large, occasionally staggering, array of details. Attending to all these details can often be done more easily and effectively by two than by one teacher. The process of coleadership of groups is the subject of the next chapter.

Appendix 4.1
Facilitating Small Group Sessions

✔ **In the groups I lead, do I...**

❑ build trusting relationships and foster collaboration?

❑ orient the learners and attend to introductions?

❑ determine the learners' experiences, needs, strengths, and
interests?

❑ help the learners understand preformulated learning goals
or develop new ones?

❑ discuss with the learners how to work together?

❑ facilitate the learners' active participation?

❑ monitor the flow of the session(s) and the group process?

❑ facilitate the flow of the session(s)?

❑ deal effectively with learners who affect the group
process negatively?

❑ deal with disagreements and manage conflicts constructively?

❑ facilitate the achievement of the members' learning goals?

❑ invite learners to process and summarize what occurs during each
session?

❑ evaluate the learners' participation and capabilities, doing what
is needed to help them and me learn from the experience?

❑ if the group meets multiple times and the members are close-
knit, prepare learners for and manage the group termination
process with care and sensitivity?

CHAPTER 5

Coleading Small Groups

In health professions education, pairs of faculty members are sometimes asked to jointly facilitate small group sessions. Educators with different backgrounds may be paired so they can complement each other's skills and perspectives. For example, a physician or nurse and a behavioral scientist might jointly teach communication skills. In groups focused on ethical issues, a clinician might be paired with a philosopher/ethicist. An interdisciplinary group (e.g., a group composed of both nursing and medical students) might be cofacilitated by a nursing educator and a medical educator.

Coleadership can take many forms. For example, during small group sessions, the cofacilitators might take turns doing tasks, such as orienting learners and providing demonstrations. Essentially one facilitator is active while the other serves as an observer or participant-observer. Or coleaders might share tasks, perhaps with one person taking the lead. One leader might introduce a new topic by presenting a case, but then the two might colead a discussion of the case. Or one might interact with the group while the other summarizes key points on a flipchart. Sometimes, in the face of busy schedules, the two leaders assigned to a group might simply take turns showing up, but that is not our focus here. Our concern is with the challenges and opportunities of working together.

Most of the principles, tasks, and strategies that apply to leading a group alone also apply to coteaching, so we don't reiterate here what we discussed in Chapters 2–4. Instead, we focus on helpful strategies that are only possible when two leaders are present. In addition, we discuss tasks and strategies that can help reduce or eliminate problems, such as coleaders trying to move the group in conflicting directions. In this chapter we discuss potential advantages and disadvantages of coleadership and examine some of the unique issues and strategies to consider when preparing for coleadership, conducting sessions, and reflecting on the effectiveness of sessions.

POTENTIAL ADVANTAGES OF COLEADERSHIP

As mentioned, leaders can share tasks (e.g., preparatory tasks, such as making certain that needed equipment is available), potentially lightening each other's load. Also, if one coleader can't attend a session, the other leader can function alone. The following points are some additional advantages of coleading small groups.

Leaders can assume complementary roles and tasks. In group leadership there are multiple tasks, some of which should occur simultaneously and are difficult for a solitary leader to do. For example, a solo leader who is interacting intensely with one member of the group can't simultaneously give adequate attention to the nonverbal behavior of the other members and may miss important cues. With coleaders, as we've indicated, one can observe while the other is engaged. The observer can then use what she learns (e.g., "John and Ruth, you looked puzzled when Dr. Tien was talking with Kevin. Do you have any questions?"). Solitary group leaders can also have difficulty focusing both on accomplishing the group's tasks and monitoring the group process, but coleaders can divide these tasks, switching back and forth as they take turns speaking. In addition, coleadership can make it possible for each leader to emphasize his or her special skills and expertise.

Learners can be exposed to different role models. To learn complex skills, such as problem solving, learners need to do more than read about them or discuss them. They need to observe professionals actually using these skills. Because there is rarely only one right way or a single optimal style for doing complex tasks, learners can be helped by observing multiple role models. For example, in a cofacilitated problem-based group, learners can observe the different ways in which their leaders approach and think through problems. In addition, the leaders can choose to highlight these differences by pointing them out (or asking learners to point them out) and discussing them.

Leaders from different disciplines can model professional collaboration. Most high-quality health care can not be provided by

practitioners functioning entirely alone, and no one professional is sufficient for the diverse and complex health needs of many patients and families. Quality care requires teamwork within and among professions. If learners are to work effectively with other health professionals, they need opportunities during their basic education to learn with representatives of these
other groups. Although on many campuses the schools of medicine, nursing, dentistry, and allied health are located near each other, few learners
have opportunitites to learn with representatives of other disciplines.

One way to foster effective interdisciplinary health care is forming
interdisciplinary student groups that are cofacilitated by educators from
the students' disciplines. Such groups can discuss topics of common interest (e.g., health care delivery) and pursue a variety of activities. If the learners
work together on health teams, they can discuss the care of their shared
patients. Even if the learners don't work together, sessions can be built
around cases prepared by faculty members in which teamwork is important. Emphasis can be placed on the complementary perspectives and roles
of the disciplines represented in the group.

***The sessions can be enriched by the coleaders' different
perspectives and leadership styles.***   Even if facilitators are from
the same discipline, they typically bring different experiences and points of
view that can help enlarge the learners' perspectives. In addition, observing and experiencing different leadership styles can help learners develop
their own leadership styles. If one of the goals of the group sessions is for
learners to develop leadership skills, attention can be drawn to the leaders'
styles and the impact of the different ways in which they present themselves and conduct the group.

Coleaders can cover each other's brief lapses.   The high level
of concentration needed for effective group facilitation can require brief
intellectual "intermissions," planned and unplanned moments of inatten-
tion during which we get some needed recuperation or reflect on some
issue, such as changes needed in the group's agenda. The presence of a
good partner, who takes over during those moments, can be a source of
considerable relief to the partner who is resting or thinking and can make
for a smoother process than solitary teachers can provide.

Leaders can learn from each other.   In most institutions, educators usually work individually with groups of students or individual learners and so are relatively isolated from one another. Cofacilitation presents
possibilities for learning about a colleague's discipline and perspectives. In

addition, cofacilitators have the possibility of observing and learning from their partner's ways of relating to and working with learners. As we indicated in Chapter 3, an effective way for inexperienced leaders (faculty members or students) to develop small group leadership skills is to be paired with experienced leaders who serve as their mentors and work with them in planning sessions and thinking through their roles and tasks. Following the small group sessions the novice leaders can reflect on and assess their efforts in the presence of their mentors and then receive feedback on the work they've done and on their self-critique. When doing so is possible, the learning can be substantially enhanced by videotaping the small group session so that the recording can be used during the review session. (If a fixed camera is used, it should be set to include the novice leader.)

POTENTIAL PITFALLS OF COLEADERSHIP

Although there are many potential advantages to coleadership, there are risks as well. If leaders don't jointly plan their sessions and come to agreement on the goals, activities, resources, and strategies, the sessions can be awkward, even chaotic. They can be negative experiences for both learners and leaders. The following are some additional potential problems that need to be anticipated so that they can be prevented.

Leaders with noncompatible or conflicting approaches to leadership and education can have difficulty working together. Even if coleaders do try planning their sessions together, if they disagree about basic issues, such as how people learn and how learning is facilitated, they are likely to have trouble devising a workable plan that is mutually acceptable. For example, if an educator who believes in and uses a collaborative approach is paired with an educator who functions in an authoritarian manner, they are unlikely to agree upon their roles and responsibilities or those of the learners and will be contradicting each other during the sessions; hardly an optimal environment for learning.

Leaders can model ineffective team behavior. Ineffective team behavior can include a variety of unappealing scenarios, including coleaders vying for power, challenging and undermining each other. When leaders are engaged in power struggles and other dysfunctional activities, they are likely to be so preoccupied with their own issues that the learners get less than they deserve.

Even potentially collaborative coleaders can take too much airtime. Many educators have difficulty suppressing their urges to talk and simply don't let learners do the amount of talking required for optimal learning. In a cofacilitated session, with the facilitators needing to share the available time for teacher talk, some educators feel even more constrained and frustrated than they would if they were leading the group alone. The competition for airtime can be aggravated if either teacher behaves, in part, out of a desire to impress his/her colleague or the students. For the sake of their learners, educators who are in intellectually competitive programs may need to work on submerging their own habits and inclinations.

TASKS AND STRATEGIES

Preparing for coleadership

Preparing for coleadership involves the same tasks as those facing solitary leaders (e.g., gathering information about learners, reviewing course materials). To some extent, though, coleaders can share these tasks. The following are some additional tasks that are unique to coleadership.

Get to know each other. The more that you know about each other, the more likely you are to be able to use each other's strengths and smoothly coordinate your efforts. If you are strangers, you might want to begin by getting to know each other as people. Also, discuss your respective views about education and about health care, as well as how you prefer approaching learners. Knowing the extent to which each of you feels you have relevant content and process skills can give you ideas about how to divide leadership responsibilities. As you get to know each other better, you can become progressively more effective as a team, even playing off each other's sense of humor and favorite stories. Many cofacilitators who are paired for the first time find that several meetings, perhaps including a meal or two, can be a worthy investment prior to their first cofacilitated group.

Share information about learners in your group. If you are from different disciplines and working with an interdisciplinary group, you will probably want to learn as much as possible about the students from each other's field (e.g., what relevant experiences they've had, where they are in their professional training). You may also want to discuss individual learners, particularly how they might contribute to the group. If there are individuals with whom you find it difficult to work, you may want to with-hold your own impressions of them, at least initially, so that your coleader's first impressions are not influenced by your opinions, unless the potential problem seems sufficiently serious to require advance planning. Seeing the learners through your coleader's eyes might help you think freshly about learners with whom you've had difficulty.

Discuss your understandings and hopes for the session.
Conflicts can develop when facilitators have different interpretations of what is expected of them by those who designed the course. Review your understandings of such factors as the purposes of the session(s), the activities in which the group is to engage, the learners' and leaders' respective roles and responsibilities, including specific tasks that need your attention. If the two of you disagree about some of these or other factors, seek information and interpretations from the course director or other sources. If you and your coleader are to make any decisions about activities, roles and responsibilities, share your ideas and try to arrive at a mutually agreeable plan.

Decide how to share leadership responsibilities. Identify
the tasks that need to be done and the skills that are needed for doing each one. Consider matching responsibilities for specific tasks with your respective capabilities, unless either of you wants to stretch yourself by doing something new.

Negotiate differences. If you appear to disagree (e.g., about how to
conduct the group, about who will do what), ensure you've heard each other clearly (e.g., by trying to summarize aloud what you thought your coleader proposed and asking your coleader to summarize what he or she thinks you are proposing). If you do disagree, consider taking turns presenting the reasons for your proposals. Try to be open to each other's proposals. Look for common concerns and interests. Look for ways in which both of you can feel good about the session(s). For example, if one of you wants the group to be structured and the other prefers that the session be unstructured, see if it's possible and educationally reasonable to have some parts of the session structured and others parts unstructured. If both of you want to do some of the same tasks and there will be several sessions, consider alternating tasks from session to session. If necessary, invite a trusted colleague to help mediate your disagreements. If all efforts to agree prove inadequate, try to arrange to change partners. Both you and your learners will likely be better off.

Table 5.1 (Sample/Partial) Plan for Group Session on Interviewing

Start time	*Activity*	*Resources needed*	*Person(s) responsible*
9:00 AM.	Introductions	Name tags	Morris
9:10 AM.	Orientation	Handouts	Chavez
9:20 AM.	Role played demonstration	Patient chart	Morris, Chavez

Develop a plan for the session. Leaders and group members can pull the group session in many different directions, and it's easy to get involved in discussions and activities and lose track of time. So, unless you are coleading a highly unstructured group, an agreed upon written session plan is key. Like session plans used by solo leaders, the plan should include the schedule, the activities, and the resources needed (see Table 5.1). Immovable times in the schedule should be noted. For example, if you know that the final activity needs 20 minutes, highlight the time when it must begin. When coleading a group, it also helps to designate which leader will have responsibility for each activity, and whether you will lead that activity alone or together.

Agree on ways to communicate with each other during sessions. If you and your cofacilitator are to succeed in steering a mutually acceptable course through the session, you have to agree that good communications between the two of you is vital, and you need to work out strategies for staying in touch during the session. Having a written plan is a good start, provided that you both use it. However, even if you are following a fairly detailed schedule, there are always multiple, moment-to-moment decisions to be made (e.g., whether to call the group's attention to a problem that is evolving, whether to linger on an unexpected, important issue even though the schedule indicates you should move on). You might know what you'd like to do, but will your coleader know what you're thinking and agree with you? Or perhaps you don't know what to do and hope your coleader has a good idea. For these and many other situations, you need to work out plans for where you will each be located in the group and how you will communicate with each other, both verbally and nonverbally.

Decide how to arrange the meeting room. The considerations for a single leader cited in Chapters 2 and 3 apply also to coleaders. In addition, coleaders need to think through where they will sit in relation to each other and the group. Some options include sitting side by side, sitting across the short end of a table from each other, and sitting at opposite ends of the room. It is usually easiest to communicate with each other if you are sitting in close proximity. If one of you tends to be a dominant leader, it is probably best not to sit at opposite ends of the room because the learners will soon have their heads turned exclusively toward the dominant leader. If you both tend to be fairly active, sitting at opposite ends can cause your group members to feel as though they are at a tennis match.

Conducting the session

As with groups led by only one leader, the tasks in a cofacilitated group include orienting learners; determining their needs, interests, and goals; clarifying preestablished goals and/or developing new ones; facilitating the active participation of all members; monitoring and facilitating the flow of the session, and more (see Chapter 4). The following are strategies that coleaders can use in accomplishing these tasks. Also we discuss some additional tasks related to coleadership.

Introduce yourselves and invite the learners to introduce themselves. Particularly if learners are not accustomed to groups with cofacilitators, include as part of your introductions an explanation about why and how you will be working together. If you and your cofacilitator are from different disciplines, this is a good time to begin conveying your respect for each other's perspectives and the rationale for bringing the two disciplines together in a learning situation. As we've said, initial impressions can have a lasting impact, so think carefully about the feeling tone you want to communicate as part of your respective introductions. Learners will quickly notice any tension, competition, or caution between you, just as they will perceive your comfort and mutual respect. After your self-introductions, invite the learners to introduce themselves, following the guidelines we presented in Chapter 4.

Model ways you want learners to interact with each other. Throughout the session you can model respect for each other, and you can model ways to ask questions, demonstrate active listening, respond to challenges, and much more. It is particularly helpful for learners to see you confront each other and deal constructively with any differences you have.

Model skills by role-playing. Besides modeling ways to function in a group, you can role-play skills students need to learn. For example, one of you can be a health professional and the other a patient, and you can demonstrate whatever skill your group is learning, such as how to explain complex information to a patient in a clear way.

Support each other's leadership efforts.   Having a supportive cofacilitator can be like having an ideal group member. If, for example, your coleader is having trouble getting a discussion started, you can begin engaging in a dialog with him and then invite others to get involved. If one of you is showing signs of fatigue, the other can step in to relieve the first person, who can relax for a few minutes.

Reinforce each other's contributions.   When your cofacilitator makes an important point, there are ways that you can reinforce what she said and demonstrate collaboration. For example, "I want to underline the importance of what Dr. Jones just said. Let me add the following example from a patient I saw recently...." If your cofacilitator is from another discipline, such reinforcement can help give him credibility with learners from your discipline.

Accommodate to a shared spotlight.   Each of you needs to be aware that your coleader will occasionally say something that you were just about to say, that students will sometimes turn to your partner when you were hoping they would turn to you, and your coleader may even be given credit for contributions that you make. You both must be comfortable that you are in a partnership and that it is your team that is at work, not two individuals. This is an accommodation that doesn't come easily to everyone. For most, it takes some time to shift from being the only teacher in the classroom to sharing leadership. So be open with your partner about the issue, and try mobilizing the patience this evolution can require.

Communicate throughout the session.   You can communicate a great deal with your coleader nonverbally. With facial expressions and gestures, you can indicate that you want to say something, or that it's time to move on to the next activity, or that you're happy or unhappy with what your coleader is doing. You can even work out gestures or hand signals for messages such as "Let's pull back and let the learners take more responsibility for this part of the session" or "Help, I don't know what to do now."

To ensure that you pick up each other's nonverbal messages, sit or stand where you can see each other and look frequently in each other's direction. Nonverbal communication can be quicker than most verbal communication, and subtle nonverbal communications can be less disruptive to the group process. There are many messages, however, that can't be adequately conveyed nonverbally. In such situations, you and your coleader can exchange notes or quietly say a few words to each other. Try not to have frequent side conversations. While you are talking with your coleader, there is a risk that you will miss what is being said, that the learners who are speaking may feel ignored, and that all members may feel excluded. To eliminate this risk, when you have something to say that is acceptable for general consumption, speak aloud to each other, preferably when there is a break in the conversation or the group reaches a branch point. For example, if your coleader is starting to move on to a new topic and hasn't checked with you to see if you're ready to make that transition, you might interrupt and say something like, "I'd like to make one comment before we move on."

If you and your coleader want learners to reflect on and feel some responsibility for the group process, address both your coleader and the group. ("Mary has been trying to say something." "We've gotten away from the topic we're suppose to discuss, but I think this conversation is so useful that I suggest we linger with it a little longer.")

Try particularly to communicate in the following kinds of circumstances:

- when you think it's time to start the session
- if you want to make a change in the agreed upon schedule or activities
- when you are taking the lead in moving on to the next activity (*To coleader*: "It's time to move on to our next activity. Do you have anything to add before we switch topics?")
- when there's a problem in the group that needs attention
- when you are unhappy with something your coleader is doing
- when it's time to switch to the session-closing activities.

Processing the sessions

Mutual critique of the session should take place as soon after each session as possible, while impressions and reactions are maximally fresh. The following are three important elements of such a critique session.

Share and compare impressions. Jointly reflecting on a group session can help you get the most possible out of the experience, and it can help you evaluate the learners' progress and the success of the session. Some questions to consider asking each other:

- How do you think it went?
- What do you think went well?
- What didn't go well? Why?
- How can we improve at the next session?

Particularly if you are expected to evaluate the learners, consider sharing your impressions of their efforts.

Critique your partnership.   Take time to reflect on how you worked together. If you will continue to work together, this step is vital. However, even if you might not work together again, doing so may give you some important insights into your leadership and coleadership approaches and skills for the future. Reflect on what went well, being as specific as possible. ("I appreciated the way you supported me when I was having trouble explaining the evaluation system.") Also, try to talk about what didn't go well. ("When you cut me off, as you did when I was trying to respond to Fred, I feel undermined as a leader.") When providing this kind of negative feedback, try adhering to these principles: be specific about events that occurred, frame your observations in terms of your feelings and perspectives, and be open to your coleader's perspective. ("This is how it seemed to me. I'd like to hear your point of view.") Since there is always room for improvement in partnerships, even if you have not had problems, try making a habit of talking with your coleader about specific ways you can improve your work together.

Critique your own efforts and provide feedback to each other.   Most of us don't get many opportunities to have our teaching observed and critiqued by peers. If you trust your coleader and feel that she can contribute to your growth, consider suggesting that you give feedback to each other. Since most of your teaching is likely done alone and you must serve as your own coach, begin these reviews with your self-critique. Then invite your coleader's critique of your self-critique, as well as her other observations and suggestions. Then switch roles.

SUMMARY

Coleaders can bring several advantages to small groups. They can learn from each other, assume complementary roles and tasks, expose learners to different role models, and provide models of professional collaboration.

They can also enrich sessions by offering different perspectives and leadership styles. Yet coleadership can also have pitfalls. Coleaders with noncompatible or conflicting approaches to leadership and education can have difficulty working together. If not appropriately prepared and skilled, they can model ineffective team behavior, and the presence of two leaders, even if they are potentially collaborative, can take too much airtime away from the learners. In Appendix 5.1 we provide a self-checklist that can serve as a summary of the special tasks involved in preparing for and implementing coleadership successfully. (For a review of the more general tasks involved in leading small groups, reread Chapters 2, 3, and 4, or at least see Appendixes 2.1, 3.1, and 4.1.)

Appendix 5.1
Special Tasks for Coleaders

✔   **Before the (first) session, did we...**

❑   get to know each other (e.g., our respective views on
        education and health care)?

❑   gather and share information about our learners (e.g.,
        relevant experiences and courses)?

❑   review our understandings and hopes for the session (e.g.,
        the goals and activities)?

❑   decide how to share the leadership responsibilities?

❑   negotiate any differences we had?

❑   develop a plan for the session(s), including our respective
        roles and tasks?

❑   agree on ways to communicate with each other during the
        session(s)?

❑   decide how to arrange the meeting room?

During the session(s), did we...

❑   introduce ourselves and invite the learners to introduce
        themselves?

❑   explain how we as leaders would be working together?

❑   model the ways that we want the learners to interact with each
        other?

❑   model skills by role-playing?

❑   support each other's leadership efforts?

❑   reinforce each other's contributions?

❑   accommodate to a shared spotlight?

❑   communicate with each other throughout the session(s)?

Appendix 5.1 (*continued*)

After the session(s), did we...

☐ share and compare our impressions/reactions?

☐ constructively critique our partnership?

☐ each critique our individual efforts and provide constructive feedback to each other?

☐ use what we learned to prepare for the next session?

2

Planning for and Leading Groups with Specific Tasks

CHAPTER 6

Facilitating Discussions and Dialogues

An intent of most small groups is providing opportunities for learners to talk with each other. Some groups, typically called "discussion groups," are devoted entirely to conversation that is intended to promote learning. David Bohm (1993), a distinguished theoretical physicist, points out that the word *discussion* has the same root as *percussion* and *concussion.*[1] In discussions, he says, the subject of common interest may be analyzed and dissected from the points of view of the participants, who thereby can learn from each other, but the purpose of discussion is often to persuade others to accept your point of view (Senge, 1990). Discussions defined this way have a place in health professions education, but what would often be more desirable is dialogue.

The word *dialogue* comes from the Greek *dialogos*. Dia means through. *Logos* means the word, or more broadly, the meaning. In dialogue, Bohm contends, the group pursues or accesses a "pool of common meaning" that is larger than what is available to any of the participating individuals. As Senge (1990) explains, in effective dialogues individuals suspend their assumptions (literally put them out front where they and others can examine them). They also moderate their certainty, becoming willing to have their thinking influenced by others. The result is an exploration that brings the participants' experiences and thoughts to the surface and goes beyond their individual views.

Ross (1994) explains that there is a continuum ranging from raw debate to polite discussion, to skillful discussion, to dialogue. The further you move toward the dialogue end of the continuum the more that attention

---

[1] The word *discussion* stems from the Latin *discutere*, which means "to smash to pieces" (Senge et al., 1994).

is paid to revealing and examining the assumptions and values behind the words that are spoken. He contends that the primary difference between skillful discussion and dialogue is intention. In skillful discussion the group intends to reach some sort of closure (e.g., make a decision, achieve agreement, identify priorities). Members may explore new issues and build deeper meaning among themselves but their intent is convergent thinking. In contrast, in dialogue the intention is exploration, discovery, insight, and a richer grasp of complex issues. The group may reach some agreement, but that isn't their primary purpose in being together.[2]

In effective discussions and dialogues, learners in the health professions are encouraged to examine their current knowledge in the areas under discussion and to build new knowledge, perhaps on a restructured knowledge base. This knowledge building occurs as they express their ideas and perspectives, try making sense of some of the volumes of information to which they are exposed, engage in collective inquiry,[3] hear the perspectives of others, reflect on new information and challenges, and constructively challenge their own and each other's assumptions and thought processes. In effective dialogue groups, learners are encouraged to elaborate on the knowledge they are building, using it in multiple ways, creating a rich web of deep connections. The learners give and take. They teach and learn. In other words, the group members engage actively in doing what is needed for meaningful, lasting learning. Rather than memorizing what they hear in lectures and read in books merely to pass exams, in dialogues learners can build their own solid, lasting knowledge bases.[4]

Discussions and dialogues are usually most effective when they are provoked by readings, presentations, observations, or other experiences that help generate interest, focus attention, and create a relevant context. (Learners will be most motivated to learn and will be most able to recall knowledge when they recognize that this knowledge is needed in their real world.) In later chapters we talk about discussions and dialogues that occur in various specific contexts. Here we discuss provoking dialogues and discussions with external events (e.g., a panel discussion, a visit to a nursing home) and/or by creating internal events (e.g., showing video triggers, read-

---

[2] Our intent in presenting this contrast between *discussion* and *dialogue* is to foster a richer understanding of the options available to us when teaching in small groups, not to encourage a preoccupation with labels.

[3] *Inquiry* comes from the Latin *inquaerere*, to seek within (Senge et al., 1994).

[4] Well more than a half-century ago Whitehead (1916) recognized the limitations of exam-oriented fact acquisition, pointing out that it leads only to "inert" knowledge.

ing poems, or doing role plays) that help establish a relevant context. Although we think that all groups should include attention to the human dimensions of learning (e.g., how learners are personally affected by the experiences in which they are engaging), we give special attention to that issue in Chapter 10 and here focus more on cognitive issues.

"Dynamic lecturers captivate a class by the virtuosity of their individual performances. Master discussion leaders accomplish the same and more by skillful guidance of the group's collective thinking process" (Lowman, 1984, p. 119). As Christensen (1991, p. 16) observed, the leader is "planner, host, moderator, devil's advocate, fellow-student, and judge — a potentially confusing set of roles." Discussion leaders face a myriad of challenges (e.g., how to get the discussion started, how to involve all learners, how to keep the discussion from being dominated by a subset of students). From moment to moment, they are faced with decisions: Is this a good time to pose a new question? Who should I call on? Should I continue my dialogue with this student or should I get the students to talk with each other? Should I answer that student's question or turn it back to her or to the group? To be effective, facilitators must recognize when such decisions are needed in the first place. Effective facilitators know that meaningful learning requires active dialogue among the learners themselves, so they retreat toward the background when appropriate, encouraging learners to engage directly with each other, coaching and supporting them only when needed.

Discussions and dialogues can have a life of their own. Although it's important to plan and prepare for discussions, it's also important to leave room for unpredictable events that can result in valuable, unanticipated learning. Christensen (1991) aptly observes that teaching in groups is the "art of managing spontaneity." Effective leaders are comfortable with, even welcoming of, uncertainty. Good discussions, Christensen adds, unfold in unexpected ways and modify the programmed logic of a teaching plan. "They pose new questions, uncover and gnaw away at sanctified assumptions, rejuvenate old topics with fresh insights, broaden perspectives, and create new paths of inquiry" (p. 106). Unlike lecturers who set and control the agenda, discussion leaders manage but don't fully control the emergence, direction, and evolution of events.

In the remainder of this chapter we identify key tasks and challenges in preparing for and conducting discussions and dialogues and offer some strategies and resources for accomplishing these tasks.[5]

---

[5] See Chapter 1 for other reasons for using discussion groups for fostering learning.

PREPARING FOR THE INITIAL SESSIONS

In Chapters 2 and 3 we presented generic leadership tasks and strategies involved in planning small group sessions. Here we expand on and supplement some of those tasks with reference to the specific situation of leading small group discussions and dialogues.

Deciding whether to engage the group in a discussion or dialogue

Think through the purposes of the group and decide which mode of communication is most appropriate or whether the group needs to do both. For example, if you want the group to think divergently, dialogue will probably be most helpful. Remember though if learners are accustomed only to conventional discussions, the group might not be able to achieve dialogue in the initial sessions or without some guidance from you.

Planning or reviewing plans for external experiences

The likelihood that a discussion or dialogue will be fruitful can be increased by having the learners begin thinking about the planned topic(s) before the session. Their thinking can be stimulated by an external experience, such as an article or story they read, a panel discussion they attend, or a field visit they undertake. To help ensure that both the external experience and the group discussion are meaningful, consider creating a framework that learners can use before and during the discussion to help them recognize how the topic is relevant to them. For example, if the topic is the pros and cons of health maintenance organizations (HMOs), you could distribute both an article that summarizes how a steadily growing proportion of graduates in their fields are being employed by HMOs and an article describing how HMOs function. You might ask learners to prepare a summary of their questions and personal conclusions to bring to the group to serve as a springboard for the discussion.

If the discussion or dialogue in your small group is to be stimulated by an external experience that has been planned by others, knowing something about that experience, even engaging in it with the learners, could enrich your planning and the discussion itself. Pay particular attention to whether the experience is being framed to help the learners recognize the linkages to what they will need to know or do as professionals. If it isn't, you may need to help students put what they hear, see, or read into a meaningful context. For example, if your small group is to discuss chronic illness but the lecture they are supposed to attend is likely to be didactic, or the article they are to read is excessively abstract, you may need to provide them with a patient case or an experience during the group that helps them make that connection. (If the external experience is not relevant, you may want to talk with the course director about ways to make it more so.) If you have access to the group members before they engage in the external experience, you can give them a framework to use and one or more tasks to do.

Planning or reviewing plans for internal experiences

You can bring life to topics and sessions and also help focus the conversation by providing learners with shared experiences during group meetings. For example, you can show them a video trigger, read a poem, present a written case history, or have them do a role play. (See Chapter 8 for a discussion of the effective uses of role plays.) Simply engaging in these activities, however, doesn't guarantee that groups will succeed. As we discuss next, careful thought needs to go into the design and selection of the resources, the timing of their use, the preparation of the learners, and the decision of what to do immediately following the activity.

Video triggers. Video triggers (vignettes) are brief (often less than 2 minutes) video clips that are intended to stimulate reactions, responses, and discussions. Typically they are segments that were specially produced or were extracted from recorded patient interviews, television programs, or films. Many video triggers are real or dramatized events (often incomplete) that are used to provoke intellectual and/or emotional reactions and stimulate discussion. Video triggers most appropriate for use with health professionals usually involve interactions between health professionals or learners and patients/clients, or between two or more health professionals.

Video triggers designed for health professionals are available through professional associations (e.g., American Psychiatric Association, Association for Surgical Education, Society of Teachers of Family Medicine) and publishers/distributors (e.g., American Journal of Nursing Company, Centre Communications, Health Sciences Consortium). If you want to create your own, the easiest way is to extract triggers from television programs (e.g., news stories, documentaries, situation comedies, and health care-oriented dramas, such as *Northern Exposure*, *ER*, *Chicago Hope*, and *911*) or films available on video that deal with issues pertinent to health professionals (e.g., *Ordinary People, Rain Man, Lorenzo's Oil, The Doctor*). Alexander, Hall, and Pettice (1994) discuss how they use clips from popular films or entire films to teach about psychosocial issues. For example, they use *The Color Purple* and *Nuts* for discussions of child abuse, *On Golden Pond* for discussions of aging, *Kramer vs. Kramer* for divorce and single parenthood, *The Dead Poets' Society* and *The Breakfast Club* for adolescence, *My Left Foot* for disabilities, and *Sleeping with the Enemy* for discussions of spouse abuse.

Television programs and films are copyrighted. As of this writing, however, the "fair use" agreement appears to permit the use of videos and films for educational events for which there is no separate charge. (You should not make copies or give them to others.) Regardless of how you use them and whether you record them off the air or purchase or rent them, we recommend talking with audiovisual experts at your institution and even seeking legal counsel to be sure you are within the law.

If you want to use a trigger (segment) from a longer tape, have the segment cued up in advance and ready to go. To use several segments from the same program, you can avoid the time-wasting process of hunting for each segment by editing the triggers onto a separate tape, leaving a couple of seconds of blank tape between each trigger. (For a fuller discussion of selecting, creating, and editing triggers, see Westberg and Jason, 1994a.)

Highlights of cases.   You can get the attention of most health professionals and health professions students by presenting relevant key features of a clinical case. Some learners become even more intrigued if the case is presented as a story in ordinary prose rather than in the cold, clinical language often used in case presentations. (In the next chapter, we discuss having learners work through cases as part of problem-based learning.)

Poems and excerpts from stories, novels, and plays.   Literature that vividly captures the experiences and values of patients, families, and practitioners as they confront illness, disability, birth, aging, and death can stimulate thoughtful conversation. For example, excerpts from Marsha Norman's play *'Night, Mother* or Albert Camus' *Plague* can provoke discussions about suffering and suicide. Tillie Olsen's "Tell Me a Riddle," Maya Angelou's "The Last Decision," and Wallace Stegner's *Angle of Repose* offer insights about aging and disability. Chronic illness can be illuminated by Ann Sexton's *The Addict* and Franz Kafka's *Metamorphosis*.

Dialogues about dying and death can be provoked by Alice Walker's short story, "Medicine," Leo Tolstoy's *The Death of Ivan Illych*, and Elie Wiesel's *Night*.[6] Autobiographical accounts of illness and caregiving can also stimulate discussion. You or others can do brief readings in class and/or learners can be asked to do some reading before coming to the group session.

Other resources.   Visitors who can present alternative perspectives and points of view can help with the tasks of focusing and stimulating dialogue. For example, a dialogue about ways to present sensitive care to the elderly can be enriched by the presence of an articulate elderly person.

Preparing yourself

Effective group leadership requires being prepared on both a cognitive and personal level. Reading and reflecting on the topics to be discussed can help with cognitive preparation, particularly if you try to put yourself in the learners' shoes as you do this reading. On a personal level, you might want to reflect on the characteristics of effective group leaders (Chapter 2) and mentally prepare yourself for areas in which you feel you are not as ready as you want to be. For example, if you decide you need to be a better listener, you could read about and practice active listening. Before walking into the group session, you could take a moment to clear your head and remind yourself to listen. As an incentive to listen, you could try anticipating the benefits of your learning from the students.

Developing a plan for the session

The elaborateness and specificity of your plan should depend on such factors as what you need to accomplish during the session and how much time you have. As we discuss in Chapter 3, if you have a lot of ground to cover in a short time, you will probably need a fairly detailed schedule. Even if the group is designed to be unstructured and freewheeling, we suggest writing down some stimulating questions that you can have in reserve to ask the group, if needed. Of course, to prepare appropriate questions, you need some initial understanding of the learners' levels of knowledge or readiness and of the key concepts you hope they will address.

---

[6] For other ideas see the collection of poetry and prose edited by Reynolds and Stone (1991), the annotated bibliography edited by Trautmann and Pollard (1982), and the literature and medicine database on the World Wide Web (http://mchip00.med.nyu.edu/lit-med/medhum.html). Also see the poems of Marilyn Krysl (1989) who spent a year in the world of nursing with faculty members, students, patients, and families. (Most of the above materials can be used by all the health professions.)

FACILITATING THE SESSION

Creating a collaborative environment

Some learners come to groups expecting a competitive event. Their mind-set is to impress their teacher and peers with what they know. As Christensen (1991, p. 19) observed, this competitive mind set can be destructive:

> When participants compete to score individual points rather than collaborate to build group themes, they damage the fabric of discussion. In such a milieu students resist modifying early conclusions even when contrary evidence emerges—a particularly dangerous practice for intellectual growth.

In competitive environments, discussions can flounder because some students are afraid to take risks for fear of publicly exposing their uncertainty or ignorance. Students who are worried about getting a good grade are likely to restrict themselves to saying only what is intended to please or impress the instructor.

If you suspect that learners are coming to the group with a competitive mind-set—that they are accustomed to "raw debate"— and you want them to listen respectfully to each other, to be open to changing their thinking, your first tasks will probably have to include inviting them to reflect aloud about the potential consequences of competitive and collaborative approaches. If you want learners to engage in the highly collaborative process of dialogue, you may need to spend even more time on these issues. In either case, be prepared to be patient.

Some learners, especially those in educational programs with traditional curricula, come to groups expecting the leader to give them "pearls." They regard discussions as merely events where people "share their ignorance." Some learners who are products of conventional programs even contend that teachers aren't doing their jobs unless they are giving students what they are expected to know. If you suspect that some members of your group hold these views, try determining if such is the case. For example, as part of the orientation you might say, "Some people think that discussions/dialogues are just times for sharing ignorance. Do any of you think that this is true?" If you discover that some learners hold this view, the first discussion you probably need to have with this group is one focused on helping them understand the reasons for discussions/dialogues. You could start by asking the group members to think of the potential advantages and disadvantages of discussions/dialogues and the potential advantages and disadvantages of traditional lectures. Be prepared with examples and arguments that can help them understand the rationale for their active involvement in thinking about and using the information they need.

The opening moments of a group are critical in setting the tone for the rest of the session. If you want learners to do their own thinking and be respectful of each other, open to alternative ideas and perspectives, willing to take risks, and eager to build knowledge together, then setting the stage for this way of working together is essential. For some suggestions of how to do this, see the section "Building trusting relationships and fostering collaboration," beginning on page 73.

Acknowledging any preparations learners made for the session

Any time that we ask learners to prepare for a group, we need to recognize what they did. Otherwise, the next time we ask them to prepare, they may not do so or may do so only halfheartedly. If learners were to read an article, go on a field visit, or prepare in some other way for the session, begin by checking on their reactions. Ask them what questions or issues emerged as they engaged in the activity. If learners have multiple questions and issues, consider writing them on a chalkboard or flipchart or asking a group member to do this. Recording their thoughts helps learners know you've heard them, and you can then review the list with the group and ask them to prioritize the questions according to how eager they are to address each one. Writing questions on a chalkboard literally keeps them in front of you and the group, and the prioritized questions can serve as an agenda for the current or some future session(s).

Doing an initial assessment

If the learners present the questions and issues that emerged for them as they prepared for the session, what they say is likely to give you some clues about their current levels of understanding of the topics in question and the extent to which they are motivated to learn more. Also be aware of the *ways* they are speaking and what may be behind the words they are saying (the "subtexts"). Are they speaking with passion or more out of a sense of obligation? Are they really curious or just trying to impress you? Are there some unspoken questions and comments that need to be brought to the surface? If you don't get the diagnostic information you need from this activity or if there was no expected preparation for the session, consider gathering such diagnostic information at the beginning of the session with direct questions to the group about the session's topics.

Initiating discussions and dialogues

The opening moments of a group, especially a new group, can be awkward. Few new instructional discussions begin spontaneously. Most need to be provoked. Here we suggest some strategies for getting discussions started effectively.

Begin with a challenge.   If the learners were given external experiences to pursue prior to the session, their questions and issues can serve as the stimulus for discussion/dialogue. If in the absence of such questions, or in addition to such questions, you plan to use a video trigger, a poem, a case, or another activity as a stimulus for discussion/dialogue, consider the following:

Set the stage.   Sometimes simply reading a poem or showing a video trigger without first preparing the learners can grab the learners' attention and stimulate their curiosity. For most material, however, it helps to set the stage first. Doing so often needs to include giving learners some background information (e.g., telling them a little about the story from which you will read a passage or the film from which you have extracted a vignette).

Give learners a challenge.   Often, the learning value of a story or video trigger is enhanced by first presenting a set of questions or other challenge that helps focus the learners' attention. ("As you watch this video trigger try to identify the ethical dilemma facing this practitioner and the family she is working with." Or, "Imagine that you are the health professional in this situation. What would you do next and why?")

Repeat the challenge.   After presenting the story or video, briefly reiterate the challenge. Learners may get caught up in the content of the presentation and forget the specifics of the challenge.

Use an open-ended approach.   As in patient care, beginning with an open-ended question encourages conversation and gives learners maximum freedom to express what they are thinking and feeling. ("What's your reaction to that poem?" "How would you describe that interaction?") On the other hand, closed questions (e.g., "Were you familiar with the poem I just read?") are likely to result in short, focused answers that can terminate rather than initiate conversation.

Encouraging learners to participate

Capturing the learners' attention is an important first step. However, to ensure that all learners, including shy and introverted students, participate, consider the following options. (See Chapter 4 for other ways to encourage participation. See also ideas for ways to keep a subset of learners from dominating the discussion, beginning on page 94.)

Wait for learners to respond. One of the major stumbling blocks to interactive conversations is teachers answering their own questions. In her studies of teachers and teaching, Rowe (1986) found that when teachers asked questions of students, they typically waited only 1 second or less for the students to reply. If students hadn't replied in that time, most teachers began offering their own response or presenting their next question. However, when the teachers increased the average length of the pauses to 3 seconds or more at two key points (after a question and after a student response), there were substantial increases in the students' participation, with pronounced positive changes in their use of language and logic. There were also positive changes in the students' and teachers' attitudes and expectations.

Some students are accustomed to teachers answering their own questions, so initially they withhold their responses. If silences are uncomfortable for you, after asking a question consider counting slowly to three or ten. If you sense that students didn't understand your question, try rephrasing it and again wait for their responses. If these extended pauses are new for you and the students, be patient. You may have to use pauses multiple times before the students are fully convinced that you truly want their participation.

Listen actively and nonjudgmentally. When learners do speak, try to put distractions and your own assumptions aside. Listen to them as openly and intently as possible, and let them know that you are listening (e.g., by looking directly at them). Try postponing your reactions to learners' statements, providing time during which you and others can reflect on what was said.

Involve multiple learners, including quiet ones. To elicit as many responses as possible, scan the group as you ask questions. Pose your questions and try not to telegraph your reaction to learners' initial responses. Be friendly but noncommittal. ("Does anyone else have another point of view?") Be careful to maintain the same neutrality when responding to both comments you agree with and those you don't, or you will unduly influence the students' participation, especially among those who want to impress or please you.

If some students are not speaking, consider looking directly at them, even giving them encouraging nods. Sometimes it helps to be more directive, particularly if more aggressive students keep cutting off quieter ones. ("Susan, you look like you have something to say." "Jorge has been trying to get in on this discussion. Let's hear what he has to say."). If, even with encouragement, a student doesn't participate, consider talking with him after the session to assess what is happening.[7]

Build what learners say into the conversation. To foster participation and collaboration, help learners see how their thoughts are contributing to the discussion. For example, use their words when possible. ("As Brian said, . . .")

Make clear that your statements are open to challenge.
If learners perceive you as credible and powerful, or they are in the habit of deferring to their teachers, they may attribute more weight to your comments and responses to questions than you want them to. By being genuinely open to other perspectives, and, emphasizing your openness, you can help reduce their inclination to be deferential. ("One approach is.... What are your ideas about other approaches?") Also avoid the kinds of absolute statements and judgmental responses that discourage disagreement or discussion.

Help learners communicate clearly

Discussions and dialogues can get bogged down when learners don't express their thoughts and feelings clearly. Since health professionals need to be clear communicators, most groups should probably include the goal of helping the learners enhance their communications skills.

---

[7] See Chapter 4 for possible reasons why learners don't participate actively in discussions or other activities.

Model patience and encourage learners to do likewise.

When learners have difficulty articulating their thoughts and feelings, other group members may get impatient and interrupt the speaker. Also, well-meaning group members may try to speak for learners who have trouble expressing themselves. When learners get impatient and interrupt, consider saying something like, "Let's give Fred a chance to tell us what he thinks." If others try to speak for a learner, nonverbally or directly communicate your desire to hear from the learner. (Gently hold up your hand to stop the interrupting learner, or say, "I'd like to hear what Fred has to say.") Allow for silence if that will help learners collect their thoughts. You might make your goal explicit by saying something like, "We all need practice toward becoming good communicators."

Ask for clarification and encourage learners to do likewise.

Some learners use language and concepts that others don't understand. Learners may also use ambiguous words or phrases that have different meanings to different people. Encourage learners to define new and ambiguous terms. Urge listeners to give feedback if they don't understand what is said. ("Can you explain what you mean by the word . . .")

Sometimes listeners can't understand speakers whose comments are muddled or irrelevant. Strategies for dealing with these challenges include nonjudgmentally letting learners know that you haven't understood them and inviting them to try again. If you still have trouble understanding them, try paraphrasing what you think they are trying to say and then check for understanding. ("Did I capture what you were trying to say?") If the points they are making seem irrelevant, consider saying something like, "Can you help me understand how what you are saying relates to our topic?" If effective communication is a learning goal for group members, it is reasonable to dwell on this process of achieving clarity and then reflect with the group on the steps involved in becoming clearer communicators. Doing this may help them develop a set of skills that can have more lasting value and importance than the information they acquire in the group.

Help learners reframe their ideas and comments.

Sometimes learners use language that disrupts rather than promotes dialogue. If learners use language that is offensive to others or unnecessarily polarizing, help them recognize the impact of what they've said. ("When you used the phrase *seductive patient*, some members of our group seemed upset. How about checking out why they reacted that way?") Invite speakers to reflect on what they mean. If appropriate, invite them to try reframing what they said so that their words foster rather than disrupt discussion.

Help learners focus.   For a variety of reasons (e.g., a tendency to talk when they're nervous), some learners disrupt discussions by presenting too many ideas at once, often meandering from one topic to another. Strategies for dealing with ramblers include interrupting them, giving them feedback, and helping them focus. For example, "Excuse me, Jeremy, but I need to interrupt you. You've already made several points. Let's deal with them before moving on to others." If you are confused by what a learner said, you might say something like, "You seem to have a number of points. Could you briefly restate the point you'd most like to make at this time." Don't hesitate to add "What can we learn about clear communication from the exchange we've just had?"

Ask learners to expand on their ideas.   Some learners speak in shorthand and don't provide enough information for others to understand them. This is particularly true of learners who don't feel entitled to airtime. Strategies for helping these learners can include giving them nonverbal and verbal messages that you want to hear what they have to say and asking them to expand on what they've said ("Could you tell us more about. . ." "Would you give us an example?"). If what they said was so abbreviated that it was incomprehensible, consider asking them to start over. ("I'm intrigued by what I think you're trying to say, but you so condensed what you said that I'm not sure I understand. Could you start over and take a little more time to explain what you mean?")

To make matters worse, some learners who speak in shorthand also speak rapidly. Sometimes it helps to interrupt them and in a friendly, caring way ask them to slow down so that you can understand them.

Some learners are too abbreviated in their statements because they are insufficiently sensitive to their hearers' perspectives. They understand their own point and assume that, therefore, everyone else must. Many learners are less sensitive to the perspectives of others than they need to be for optimal communication, so drawing explicit attention to this issue and spending some time dealing with it can make a valuable contribution to their growth.[8]

---

[8] This discussion of helping learners enhance their communication skills assumes that you are open to reflecting on and, if needed, refining your own skills. As with any skill, to be

Helping learners be aware of and examine their understandings, assumptions, and values

A common reason for learners not being able to communicate clearly is that they are not clear about what they think. Conventional education in which learners try to memorize the thinking of others rather than build their own knowledge can leave learners with unrecognized and unexamined assumptions, beliefs, and values. Learners may even be left with little confidence in their ability to think for themselves.

As learners engage in the kinds of effective external and internal activities we've described, they may become aware of understandings they didn't realize they had. They may conclude that their current understandings are adequate for the challenges they face, or they may decide their understandings are incomplete or insufficient. Such cognitive conflicts can motivate people to learn (Fosnot, 1989). As we've indicated and discuss later, exposing learners to multiple points of view can present them with useful contrasts and constructive challenges to their thinking. The following are some other strategies to use.

Encourage learners to voice their thoughts. The act of trying to articulate their understandings can help learners be more self-aware. Most of us have experienced the phenomenon of thinking that we know and understand something...until we try explaining it to others. It is only then that we may realize how shallow our understanding really is. Also, the nonverbal and verbal feedback learners who are voicing their thoughts get from their peers can help. For example, a learner may re-examine her belief that her thinking is clear if group members indicate they can't understand her. In addition, if other learners challenge what she says, she may reach greater clarity, particularly if she is open rather than defensive. (Learners are most

---

helpful to others, you need to understand the elements of that skill and be able to serve as a role model of its implementation. For example, if you are unfamiliar with the concept of "subtext" or are not accustomed to reflecting on your ways of communicating and your impact on others, consider reviewing the section (p. 138,) "Helping Learners Communicate Clearly," focusing on the examples of comments you might make in groups. Try saying some of those statements out loud, using contrasting forms of emphasis, facial expression, and body language, challenging yourself to cause these same words to have a positive and then a negative impact on imaginary listeners. Remember, listeners pay even more attention to your *ways* of communicating than to the words you use. If you are serious about enhancing your skills as a communicator, consider setting up a home camcorder for recording and then reviewing this practice of alternative ways of communicating. Or join a faculty development workshop where you can get both practice and constructive feedback on your communication skills.

likely to be open if their peers offer challenges and feedback in constructive ways, as we discuss later.)

Help learners examine what is behind what they say. A statement that a learner makes may or may not be the result of systematic thinking on his part. (The statement could be based on something he read or heard but has not yet assimilated.) Also, he may or may not be aware of assumptions and values that underlie his (or his source's) conclusions. Sometimes the way learners present an idea provides a clue. (If the idea is not the learner's, she may present it incoherently. If the statement is based on a strongly held value, she might make a statement with some passion or uncompromising assertiveness.) At other times, though, you may need to do some probing before you can be certain. Some questions that can help you get below the surface include[9]

- Could you explain how you arrived at that conclusion?
- What do you mean by . . .?
- What are your reasons for thinking this is so?
- How do you know that that's true?
- If what you suggest is true, then how would you explain. . .?

If you want to help learners be aware of and examine their assumptions or values, try being direct. ("Are you aware of any assumptions you are making?" "Are you aware of any ways your conclusion might be shaped by your values?") If your learners are not accustomed to thinking in these terms, you might need to start with a more basic discussion of what assumptions and values are and how they can influence one's thinking.[10]

Encouraging active listening

True dialogue cannot occur without active listening. One of the most frequent complaints among group members is that they do not feel they are fully heard by others (Goldberg & Larson, 1975). Their questions remain unanswered; their ideas are ignored. The group conversation is disjointed and disconnected.

---

[9] As you read each of these questions, consider saying them out loud in two different ways: (1) neutrally and inquisitively, and (2) harshly and judgmentally. We trust you will want to consistently use the first approach.

[10] We're not suggesting that you reserve this probing approach only for learners who you suspect have not carefully thought through issues for themselves. Raising these kinds of questions with all learners can help them develop the valuable intellectual habit of routinely asking these questions of themselves.

In an investigation of communication in effective and ineffective groups, Evelyn Sieburg examined the ways members responded to the communicative acts of others. In this study and in other work with Carl Larson (Sieburg & Larson, 1971), Sieburg identified responses that she classified as confirming or disconfirming. Disconfirming responses that blocked communication include:

- ignoring or disregarding other speakers' attempts at communication
- interrupting others, by cutting them off or starting to talk before they have finished
- responding in a way that seems unrelated to what the other has been saying or introducing a new topic or returning to an earlier topic, apparently disregarding the intervening contribution
- acknowledging the other person's communication but immediately taking the conversation in another direction
- responding in an incoherent way (e.g., with sentences containing much retracing or rephrasings).

We can add reading, sleeping, and cross talking while a member is trying to speak with the group. A major cause of nonattention to what others say is our common tendency to be preoccupied with thinking about what we want to say next, while others are speaking.

Model desirable behaviors. To help learners become more active listeners, you can model the three confirming responses identified by Sieburg:

- directly acknowledging the other's (the learner's) communication
- asking for clarification when needed; encouraging learners to say more
- reinforcing information expressed by the learners.

Ask learners to paraphrase what others have said. You can help learners practice active listening by asking them to paraphrase what others say. You can also model paraphrasing yourself: "I want to be sure I understood what you were telling us, Donna. Let me try restating what you said."

Ask learners to listen to the group and report on what they hear. If you suspect that learners are not listening carefully to each other, consider asking them, one at a time, to listen and not speak for a period (perhaps 5 minutes) and then summarize what they've heard.

Encourage learners to identify barriers to their hearing others. Learners' assumptions and beliefs, particularly those that are strongly held, can limit what they are capable of hearing and seeing. If learners are having trouble hearing, explore with them the possibility that their assumptions or beliefs are getting in the way. (As teachers we all need to be doing this regularly ourselves.)

Fostering conversations among learners

Initially many learners are likely to direct questions and comments to the leader rather than to each other, making the conversation look like a spoked wheel, with the leader at the hub. Sometimes that's appropriate, but, as we've discussed, lasting learning is more likely when the learners are active participants, communicating directly with each other. Also, there are important lessons to be learned from learners assuming responsibility for the success of the discussion/dialogue. To encourage active exchanges among group members, consider using the following strategies.

Make conversations among learners an expectation. Explicitly talk with learners about the expectation that they will talk among themselves as well as with you. If they don't understand why you want to do this, discuss the rationale and provide examples.

Use "buzz groups." Particularly if the group is large and some learners are reluctant to speak, consider inviting them to briefly discuss a question or issue in subgroups of twos or threes. Many learners find it easier to speak in such buzz groups. Then, having spoken, they can feel more confident speaking to the entire group. (Sometimes after hearing each other's ideas in the buzz group, peers encourage each other to speak up in the full group.)

Invite learners to redirect their questions and comments. There are times when it's appropriate to respond directly to questions or make comments. If, however, you are trying to get learners to engage directly with each other, there are steps you can take. For example, when learners ask you a question, make a nonverbal gesture (e.g., extend your hand in the direction of the other group members) to indicate that you'd like others to respond or voice your request. ("Please ask the others what they think.")

Remain silent even when you're eager to speak. When learners are struggling with a concept that we feel we could explain to them clearly, it's very tempting to step in and straighten them out. Yet we know that students usually learn best by making their own discoveries. Sometimes, especially if there is limited available time, a quick intervention can help. If you do intervene, rather than providing an answer, try starting with a question that will help guide their thinking. Then, if necessary, make a statement.

Pull back from the dialogue. If learners keep turning to you with their questions or look to you for approval after they've spoken, consider averting your eyes (e.g., look down or scan the group) or placing your chair where you can't easily be seen by the group, particularly by members who keep looking at you. Even consider leaving the room for part or all of a session, or talk with the learners about what's happening, how you feel, why you feel as you do, and what you propose should be done about the situation.

Helping learners consider multiple points of view

Health professionals need to be able to consider and respond to other points of view, both objectively and subjectively. However, learners who are accustomed to being spoon-fed often want to be given the "right" answer and don't want to be burdened with other points of view. Conflicting viewpoints seem distracting and confusing. Group members who are afraid of conflict are prone to engaging in "groupthink" (Janis, 1972). In addition, many learners are unfamiliar with or unaccustomed to subjective thinking. Some learners are uncomfortable with or even threatened by other ways of thinking and may even act in antagonistic ways toward the bearers of other perspectives. The following are some strategies for dealing with such challenges.

Help learners value intellectual and attitudinal diversity.
To set the stage for helping learners value diverse viewpoints and perspectives, consider using the introductions as a time to get to know something about each person's background. If appropriate, express how you anticipate that the members' different backgrounds and outlooks will make the discussion richer. Consider giving the group an example from their professional world in which a team of professionals with multiple perspec-

tives solved a problem or accomplished a feat that would probably not have been possible for a person working alone. Help members recognize when their own diversity is enriching the group discussion.

Encourage learners to present alternate points of view.
Elicit diversity within the group. For example, after a student states her point of view say something like, "Does anyone have another way of looking at this issue?" Stay neutral as you collect different points of view. If the group appears to be of one mind, consider asking members to argue points of view that differ from their own. ("If you were on the opposite side of this discussion, what points would you make?") To help them gain a fuller understanding of other points of view, invite them to imagine that they are a person with another point of view. Ask them how they might feel, how they might defend that point of view, how they might react to challenges to their (adopted) points of view.[11]

Encourage learners to elicit other points of view.
As members of health teams, learners need to value and draw on the perspectives of colleagues. You can help learners practice doing this with such questions as, "Why don't you find out what other people think?" If learners elicit views from others but don't do so in an in-depth way, you can raise questions: "Do you think you understand what Tom is saying? Is there anything else you'd like to ask him?"

Raise unspoken points of view.
If points of view that you consider important don't emerge from the group, consider raising them yourself, even being a devil's advocate. ("What about . . . . ?") To help learners consider additional perspectives, use resources (e.g., poetry, film) that present other perspectives or invite to a session a visitor with a fresh point of view.

---

[11] Throughout their careers, health professionals need to be able to examine different points of view in two rather distinct ways. The first, which Belenky and colleagues (1986) call *separate knowing*, involves responding to alternative viewpoints critically and analytically. In discussion groups, learners are often encouraged to engage in such objective, analytical thinking. The second, more subjective approach, which Belenky and colleagues call *connected knowing*, is seldom encouraged and is even actively discouraged in some health professions education traditions. It is a way of thinking that's essential to providing sensitive health care. In working with patients and colleagues, health professionals need to be able to suspend their own views temporarily and try seeing the world as others see it. Effective discussion groups, in which learners are able to express their intellectual and attitudinal diversity, are good arenas for practicing both types of thinking. In addition being open to and aware of different ways of thinking can help prepare learners for dealing with the increasingly diverse, controversy-filled world of health care.

Creating an environment in which learners can take risks

Effective learners (and teachers) consider everything as open to being questioned, even what currently is regarded as truth. Such a questioning posture can fuel their learning for the rest of their lives. Creating a safe environment makes it possible for learners to raise bold questions and also take other risks. Some strategies for creating such an environment follow.

Model risk taking.   Revealing our areas of certainty and uncertainty, our hopes, and our defeats can help promote openness in students. Consider asking the group some of your own unanswered questions. Admit when you don't know an answer. Encourage learners to do likewise.

Support learners who take risks.   It is especially important to support learners who challenge popular points of view or bring up unpopular perspectives. As Christensen (1991, pp. 20–21) observed:

> If we want our students to take the risks that make creativity possible, we must show we are willing and able to assist them when they stumble. To make independence practical and enfranchise all the members of the group, we must support students when their comments depart from the consensus of the moment or their proposals collide with firmly held convictions of the class.

Support can take the form of a public statement: "Tom, I appreciate the way you've stood up for your point of view, even though what you are saying isn't popular in the group."

Help learners be critical of ideas, while not rejecting their authors.   If learners don't seem to understand that it is possible to express disagreement without attacking or rejecting others, talk with them about this concept. If they make rejecting statements or put down other learners, intervene if necessary. Help them see what they've done and reflect on what it is like to have that done to themselves. Help them rethink, rephrase, and practice alternative comments.

Probing the learners' understandings

Guiding the discussion in fruitful directions requires being continually diagnostic, not only at the opening of the session. You can be diagnostic by posing occasional questions, listening carefully to the learners' responses, and observing their nonverbal communication.

When seeking to be diagnostic, too many teachers ask fact-focused questions. When the student gives the "correct" response, however, all that the teacher has determined is that the learner was able to recall—or stumble upon—the fact, at that moment. Without further inquiry, the teacher can't know whether the answer was a lucky guess, was arrived at through a series of mutually compensating incorrect assumptions and deductions, or whether a slight variation in the terms of the question could still be handled satisfactorily by that student.

Probing understanding and challenging assumptions can be helpful to learners in multiple ways. How many times have we heard grateful students refer to instructors who "really made me think"? Asking questions that test the reasoning behind responses helps learners get in touch with what they know (and perhaps didn't even know they knew) and what they don't yet know. Asking probing questions can also help them be more careful and critical in their thinking, especially if you routinely raise these kinds of challenges, both when students appear to understand what they are talking about and when they don't.

Fostering expansive, higher-level thinking and discussion

Ask more divergent than convergent questions.   Divergent questions (e.g., "What are some other ways to handle this situation?") invite expansiveness in thinking. They require reflection, speculation, analysis, and/or reasoned conclusions. Convergent questions, on the other hand, demand a narrowing of perspective. Often they are "guess what I'm thinking" questions. In other words, they require a specific response that the teacher considers to be the one, acceptable, "right" answer. ("What is the appropriate test in this situation?")

Ask higher-level questions.   The cognitive level of teachers' questions appears to correlate significantly with the cognitive level of their students' responses (Foster, 1981). Learners are unlikely to demonstrate higher-level thinking skills (e.g., analysis, synthesis, and evaluation) when teachers ask only lower-level questions, particularly questions directed at the recall of knowledge (Centra & Potter, 1980). As you pose questions to learners, and as you help them pose questions to themselves and each other, try keeping the discussion at the higher levels of thinking that they will need to engage in as professionals.

Foster creative thinking. Critical thinking should not obliterate creative thinking. Some of the greatest advances in health care have come when practitioners or scientists have abandoned traditional, conventional, even logical thinking and have drawn upon intuition and inspiration. In speaking about his experience in a tutorial group at Harvard, a student remarked, "How refreshing to let our minds run free. There wasn't the pressure of learning to know the right answer. Instead we were encouraged to think and be creative—to use what little we did know in order to learn more" (Strayhorn, 1973). Students need to spend some of their time imagining and speculating.

Invite learners to elaborate and make connections

As we've discussed, learners are more likely to remember and use information if they have an opportunity to elaborate on this knowledge at the time of learning. This elaboration, according to Norman & Schmidt (1992), can be fostered by engaging in discussions, answering questions, or using the new knowledge when trying to understand or solve a problem. There is evidence that successful clinical reasoning is dependent on having access to "an appropriate structured memory comprising a deep, rich knowledge" (Coles, 1991). Put another way, merely being exposed to or memorizing information is insufficient preparation for later putting that information to use when needed in the real world. We don't truly possess knowledge, we don't have it functionally available for practical applications until we've used it in multiple ways. We need to have integrated it into a web or pattern of connections with our current knowledge patterns for it to become available later in the unpredictable variety of situations in which it might be needed. Discussion/dialogue groups can provide the repeated opportunities that learners need for putting new knowledge to use, for elaborating it, for making it their own.

Helping learners think together

Bohm (1993) points out that in many groups people do not think together. Rather, each person tries primarily to get his or her ideas across. However, when groups enter into true dialogue, ideas are offered, picked up, passed around. Each individual's contributions gets to be enriched by the perspectives and contributions of others. The fully elaborated ideas and understandings that emerge come to belong primarily to the group, less to individuals. When an appropriate atmosphere has been fostered in a group, the sense of individual possessiveness diminishes or disappears. This kind of collaborative group thinking is needed on health teams, where team members should be focusing primarily on the needs of their patients, less on fulfilling their own needs for recognition.

Helping learners digest what they're hearing

Elaborating and making connections helps learners build solid frameworks of knowledge. So can moments of silence, though in many discussion groups there are no such quiet times because members or the leader typically rush to fill the silences. When engaged in meaningful dialogue, Native Americans, Quakers, and other groups allow for intermittent moments of silence. In fact, during business meetings and other events, Quakers often request a few moments of silence, especially when a difficult issue has been introduced. Pauses after people speak can enable listeners to reflect more deeply on what was said, build on what they were thinking and, perhaps, link what they've just heard to what they know. Silences can enable people to gather their own thoughts instead of speaking impetuously, without reflection. And silences can open people to unexpected fresh ideas and perspectives. When Native American elders say "We will speak of this again," they recognize that meaning can develop in silence.

If your learners aren't accustomed to silence, you may need to discuss its value and use. In addition, you might indicate that once or twice during each session you will ask for silence and that students can use that time in quiet reflection, perhaps making notes for themselves. Introducing such moments for reflection into your groups can make a more general contribution to your learners. Many learners in the health professions spend so much of their time feeling under pressure that they abandon any inclination they had toward being reflective. Yet, being reflective is fundamental to being a mature professional.

Acknowledging feelings

Some health professions educators tend to ignore students' (and practitioners' and patients') feelings—to act as if feelings don't exist. Yet lasting learning isn't something that just happens intellectually. It affects one's whole being. If we want students to become compassionate, skilled health professionals, their education must engage both their heads and their hearts. For example, we can ask them to reflect on their personal reactions to and feelings about the topics under discussion. Also, even when focusing on topics that are typically discussed only in objective terms (e.g., respiratory physiology), we can elicit students' reactions to (and reveal our own enthusiasms about) the beauty and complexity of the human body. In Chapter 10, we discuss ways to help learners become aware of and deal with their feelings.

Monitoring and facilitating the flow of the session

In Chapter 4, we discussed serving as a participant-observer, both participating in the discussion and witnessing its process. Being a participant-observer enables us to consider using the following strategies.

Invite group members to reflect on what's happening. If you want the group to begin taking responsibility for the discussion, you can interrupt the conversation occasionally during the session and invite the members to summarize the exchange. ("What issues have we discussed so far?") In addition, you may want the group to "map" their discussion by having one member make a running list on a chalkboard or flipchart of topics and issues being discussed so that everyone can see the sequence as it emerges. Depending on the purposes of the group, you can also invite the learners to reflect aloud on their observations about the group's interactions. These pauses for reflection are usually best done when discussions of a topic are winding down and it is time for a transition.

In addition to pausing occasionally for content summaries, you might choose to stop the group at critical decision points or during process difficulties (e.g., when the conversation is going off target, the discussion is bogged down, or a conflict is emerging between group members) and ask them to reflect on what's happening. Remember that the act of asking the group to pause may or may not be beneficial. If appropriately chosen, an interruption can provoke the group into recognizing that they are having a problem, such as going off target, and they will get back on course, or solve whatever other problem exists. If, however, the interruption is not well timed, it can disrupt the group's energy and frustrate the learners. In other words, pausing for reflection is not a strategy to be used indiscriminately.

Share your observations with the group. You can also choose to share with the group your observations about their progress and process, either with or without first asking them for their observations. Try to make your observations specific, descriptive, and nonjudgmental. If your observation is distinctly subjective, label it as such. ("I'm running out of energy around this issue. What about the rest of you?") See Chapter 4, page 92, "Provide feedback to the group."

Intervene.   Particularly when groups are new and members are not yet ready to facilitate and monitor the group process, you may choose to be more directive. If, for example, the discussion seems to be bogging down, you may infuse it with new energy by raising an intriguing question, making an intellectually provocative statement, or showing a video trigger. If the group seems to have reached closure about a topic, you may point this out and ask them if they'd like to move to another topic. If the group needs to cover certain topics within a limited time, you, with or without the help of group members, might make a tentative plan regarding how much time to spend on each topic and then watch the clock to ensure that the discussion is moving along at an adequate pace.

Reaching closure

Particularly when the group is engaged in a lively discussion/dialogue, it can be tempting to just let the conversation flow until the end of the period. However, without time near the end for summarizing, for reflecting on what was accomplished and making follow-up plans, students can feel that the conversation is left dangling, be unclear about what was accomplished, or not know what they are supposed to do next. Thus the lasting value of their interchange is likely to be less than it might have been.

In many sessions, it's not possible to respond fully to every learner's questions or to reach satisfactory conclusions about every topic of discussion. Indeed, it can be desirable for students to leave with questions they want to pursue and ideas they want to continue exploring. However, it is possible and desirable to summarize what was accomplished, acknowledge lingering questions and unsettled issues that the group wants to pursue, and make plans for the next session or activity. As we suggested in Chapter 4, most group sessions are enhanced by taking these steps to bring closure to the event.

SUMMARY

Effective discussions/dialogues are opportunities for learners to become aware of and test their understandings, assumptions, and values, and to build rich, deep knowledge. This meaningful learning happens as learners present their thinking to others, get challenges and feedback from others, explore multiple points of view objectively and subjectively, and practice using new information in many different ways. In the self-checklist in Appendix 6.1 we summarize some of the main tasks involved in facilitating small group discussions/dialogues effectively. (For a review of the more general tasks involved in leading groups, please see Appendixes 2.1, 3.1, and 4.1.)

Appendix 6.1
Planning and Facilitating Discussions/Dialogues

✔   **Did I...**

When preparing for groups

❑   plan or review plans for external experiences for the learners
       (readings, lectures, panel discussions, field trips) that were
       intended to help stimulate discussion/dialogue?

❑   plan or review plans for internal experiences for the learners
       (video triggers, readings, case histories, role plays) that were
       intended to help stimulate discussion/dialogue?

❑   prepare myself (intellectually and emotionally)?

During the session

❑   create a collaborative environment?

❑   do an initial assessment of the learners' levels of readiness and
       acknowledge any preparations they made for the session?

❑   initiate the interchange with an engaging, relevant challenge and
       use mainly open-ended questions and comments?

❑   encourage learners to participate (e.g., by allowing enough "wait
       time" when learners or I asked questions; listening actively
       and nonjudgmentally and encouraging learners to do like-
       wise; keeping the conversation from being dominated by a
       subset of learners; building what learners said into the dis-
       cussion; making clear that my statements were open to being
       challenged)?

❑   help learners communicate clearly (e.g., by asking for clarifica-
       tion and encouraging learners to do likewise; helping learn-
       ers reframe their ideas and comments when needed; helping
       learners focus or expand their ideas, as needed)?

❑   help learners be aware of and examine their understandings,
       assumptions, and values?

❑   encourage active listening (e.g., by asking learners to paraphrase
       and identify barriers to their hearing others)?

Appendix 6.1 (*continued*)

❑ foster dialogue among the learners (e.g., by being silent even when I was eager to speak)?

❑ help learners consider multiple points of view (e.g., by helping them value diversity and present and elicit alternative points of view; by raising unspoken points of view)?

❑ create an environment in which the learners felt they could take risks (e.g., by modeling risk-taking; supporting learners who took risks; helping learners be critical of ideas not people)?

❑ probe the learners' understandings and foster higher-level thinking and discussion?

❑ invite the learners to elaborate, make connections, and think together?

❑ help the learners digest what they were hearing (e.g., by using silence)?

❑ acknowledge the learners' feelings and my feelings?

❑ monitor and facilitate the flow of the session?

❑ help the group reach satisfactory closure, as needed?

CHAPTER 7

Facilitating Problem-Based Learning Groups

In conventional classrooms, learners are introduced didactically to a discipline (e.g., physiology, biochemistry) and to topics within that discipline. Later learners may be given problems to solve. (These problems only seldom relate to the real tasks faced by health professionals.) The content of the discipline and its structure drive the instructional approach. Learners are expected to organize what they learn around the vocabulary, definitions, lists, taxonomies, and hierarchies associated with an individual discipline's subject matter. Not surprisingly, clinical teachers often complain that learners cannot access the knowledge to which they were exposed in the basic sciences when they need it in clinical situations.

By contrast, in the problem-based learning (PBL) approaches discussed in this chapter,[1] learning begins with and is stimulated by problems and challenges, particularly ones that are relevant to what the students are likely to encounter in their work as health professionals (e.g., a patient or community health problem). As in the real world, these problems can be complex and multifaceted and not confined to the artificial boundaries of a single discipline.[2] To address these problems, students—even those in the first weeks of their professional education—engage in some of the steps they will use when solving problems as professionals (e.g., generating hypotheses about what might account for a presenting problem). As they

---

[1] Problem-based learning takes many forms. The approach described here began in the late 1960s in the health sciences at Michigan State University (where it was called "focal problem teaching") and at McMaster University.

[2] The organizational structure of the "basic science" disciplines is widely acknowledged to be increasingly outdated, even for the research that is their primary reason for being. They were never organized with the intent of serving the educational needs of health professionals.

cooperatively address problems, learners, facilitated by a teacher (tutor[3]), first draw on and test what they already know. (Collectively, even beginners often have an impressive range of relevant knowledge.) When the learners find that their current knowledge falls short of what they need, like professionals who are effective learners, they identify and prioritize their learning issues,[4] identify sources for obtaining needed information, and decide who will pursue which learning issues. After obtaining new information (e.g., by reading, consulting with others) the learners share what they've learned, evaluate their sources of information, and try using their new information in explaining the case at hand. They may even solve some or all of the problems presented by the case,[5] and they may go through this learning cycle multiple times.

In other words, in well-designed PBL the ways learners approach and solve problems, and the ways they acquire and organize knowledge, parallels what they will need to do as professionals. These activities give them practice in approaching and solving problems, being self-directed, and participating in the process of collaborative learning. Engaging in these tasks can also help ensure that what they learn will be available to them when they need it later in real professional situations (Norman & Schmidt, 1992). In addition, students who consistently learn in this way during their basic education are more likely to see potential learning opportunities in every patient encounter and to engage in reflection, inquiry, and self-directed, collaborative learning throughout their careers.[6]

The educators' tasks in PBL typically include ensuring that the case is appropriate, introducing learners to the process, if needed, and guiding them through the process with questions, feedback, and other strategies that we will describe shortly. Teachers may or may not be content experts in the areas addressed in the case. (Discussions can be sufficiently wide-ranging to exceed many teachers' areas of expertise.) Even if teachers are content experts, it's generally most helpful if they use their knowledge for

---

[3] The term commonly used for those who facilitate PBL groups.

[4] In some programs (less desirably, we think) the faculty identify some or all of the learning issues.

[5] Learners can also feel good about and have fun working on solving problems. Sometimes, however, faculty members don't intend for students to solve the problem or even fully understand the underlying anatomical, physiological, behavioral, or biochemical mechanisms involved. Rather, the problem serves as a challenge to their reasoning or problem-solving skills and as an organizer for their subsequent learning.

[6] See Chapter 1, beginning at page 5, for a fuller rationale for learning in small groups.

facilitating the students' learning, rather than for giving them answers.[7]

Although a variety of different kinds of problems, queries, and puzzles are used in PBL, here we focus on clinical cases, especially those built on patient stories. Currently much of PBL in the health professions is used with students who are early in their basic professional education and who have had little or no clinical experience. The approach is used to help them acquire knowledge (particularly in the biological sciences) in the context of patient cases. However, PBL has been used to help learners at all levels of professional education, including continuing education, build knowledge.

Much has been written about PBL. In this chapter our intent is to provide only a brief introduction to what PBL is and how this approach can be used constructively in single class sessions or in a series of small group sessions. Excellent resources (e.g., Barrows & Tamblyn, 1980; Barrows, 1985, 1988, 1994; Boud & Feletti, 1991) are available for readers who want a fuller discussion of PBL, including the many forms it can take, strategies for developing entire courses or curricula in problem-based format, and strategies for introducing it into schools and programs.

In the remainder of this chapter, we identify key tasks in preparing yourself for and conducting PBL format small groups and some strategies for accomplishing these tasks.

PREPARING FOR LEADING
PROBLEM-BASED LEARNING GROUPS

In Chapters 2 and 3, we presented generic tasks and strategies involved in planning and conducting small group sessions. Here we focus on tasks that are unique or especially pertinent to PBL.

Selecting or designing cases

Cases that have been well thought out and carefully designed are key to effective PBL. There is a growing library of problems/cases suited for PBL

---

[7] If the premise that our instructional task is primarily to guide the learners' own explorations, rather than to feed them information, is new to you or hard to understand, try reflecting on your contrasting experiences of being driven around a city that's new to you (being passive) versus finding your own way (being active). People can be passengers multiple times on the same route and never learn to find their own way even if they were trying.

that can be acquired or purchased from institutions with extensive experience in developing such cases.[8] In many schools, teams of teachers develop cases together. For example, a case designed to help students learn biological sciences within a clinical situation might be collaboratively developed by clinicians, basic scientists, and an education specialist.

If you want to write a case and cannot secure advice on how to do that at your school, consider reading Hafler (1991) and Barrows (1994) and contacting colleagues in other institutions who have designed successful cases. Also, consider doing as many others have done: develop the PBL paper-based case from a real case or a composite of real cases, being careful of course to protect the privacy of the real patients.

Whether you are designing a problem package or using one that was designed by others, the following questions encompass many of the characteristics of effective cases.

Does the case cover the areas you want learners to explore? Even if you don't divulge the learning goals directly to the learners but allow the goals to emerge from the learners' experiences working on the assigned case, you still need to be clear about your goals and ensure that the case you select or devise is an appropriate vehicle for achieving and is consistent with these goals.

Does the case confront the students with challenges they are likely to encounter in the real world? Students typically work hardest on and learn most from problems they feel are realistic and they can anticipate facing.

Is the case sufficiently focused? Real patient cases can range from simple to highly complex. Hafler (1991) reported that experienced case writers at her school had concluded that cases should have a central topic or theme, similar to a mystery story, rather than multiple themes. She also said that "red herrings" could be appropriate for advanced students but seldom for first-year students.

Is the case appropriate for the learners' levels of knowledge? Barrows (personal communication, 1995) is persuaded that tutors and groups can make virtually any problem appropriate for the full range of learners, from first-year students to experienced practitioners, by deciding which aspects of the problem to tackle. Norman and Schmidt (1992) argue that

---

[8] For example, McMaster University Schools of Medicine and Nursing, Southern Illinois University School of Medicine, and the University of New Mexico School of Medicine.

problems are best when an in-depth understanding is beyond the learners' current knowledge when first encountered.

Does the case provide the learners with practice in gathering information and solving problems as they would in real-life situations? Currently the term *PBL* is used to refer to a wide variety of educational practices that use different kinds of problems (Boud & Feletti, 1991). In part, the problems differ in the extent to which they present and unfold like they would in the real world and in the extent to which they are designed for learners to take the kinds of actions they would need to take in the real world (e.g., information gathering, hypothesis testing). Barrows (1986) describes three major types of problems:

1. *Full problem simulations* are the most realistic. Learners are given the kind of unorganized information they would initially encounter in the real world. For example, learners might be given a written paragraph containing some relevant and even irrelevant information, such as they might gather in the first few minutes of a patient visit. Or learners might gather the initial information themselves (e.g., by interviewing a standardized patient—a person who is trained to present with certain problems, symptoms, feelings, and life situations). After reflecting on this initial information, learners gather further information through free inquiry (e.g., by continuing to interview the patient, or by questioning their tutor) . They may also be given some updates on the problem situation.

2. *Complete cases* are organized summaries of key facts that the writer(s) of the problem decided learners needed to know. The learners' task is to figure out what may be going on with the patient and what to do next.

3. *Partial problem simulations* are compromises between the first two types of problems. For example, patient management problems (PMPs) (McGuire, Solomon, & Bashook, 1976) might begin in a realistic way, but the actions that learners can take are typically restricted to the options that are presented.

Is the problem real and "ill-structured"? Barrows (1994) argues that effective problems should have the characteristics that cognitive psychologists call being *ill-structured.* In such problems

1. more information is needed for understanding the problem than is immediately available

2. there is no one right way to get the information; the problem solver has to question, explore, observe, probe, and experiment to get further information
3. the understanding of the nature of the problem often evolves and changes as new information is acquired
4. the problem solver cannot be sure the analysis of the problem, the solution, or the action taken to resolve the problem is definitively the right one (p. 10).

In contrast, Barrows points out that only in textbooks or poorly designed classroom cases does one find problems in which all the information needed to work on the problem is available, the method to use for solving the problem is defined, and the learners get a clear indication of whether the problem has been correctly solved or managed. Such "clean" problems are not reflective of and not optimal preparation for the real world.

Does the case capture the human dimensions and the context of the problem(s)? Naming (not with real names, of course) and describing the people in the cases and including psychosocial, cultural, ethical, and spiritual factors can help the scenario come alive and enhance the learners' understandings of the multidimensional, wholistic nature of real clinical work. Ensuring that the people in the cases represent both genders and a range of races, cultures, and ages, as well as socioeconomic and educational backgrounds, can help prepare learners for working sensitively with the diverse populations they are likely to face later.

Deciding how learning issues will be generated

At some schools student-generated objectives are the key focus for learning. Students take responsibility for determining what needs to be learned, how it is to be learned, and at what pace (Wilkerson, Hafler, & Liu, 1991). At other schools students use faculty-generated learning objectives with reading assignments to guide their learning of basic science concepts. At still other schools, students are able to see faculty objectives after they have generated their own, or their tutors may have a handbook listing the objectives that they can use in guiding discussions (Blumberg, Michael, & Zeitz, 1990). Factors to consider when deciding what to do include the amount of support you think learners need, the context in which your small group session is taking place, and the amount of time available. Ask yourself what will potentially be gained and lost if students generate some or all of their own learning issues.

Deciding on resources and strategies to use in presenting the case

If you are creating your own case, or creating it with others, there are a number of resources and strategies to consider using when presenting the case to learners. You might also want to consider using some of these resources and strategies to enliven any cases you use that were prepared by others.

A written document. Many teachers give the learners a written document. It can be as simple as one or two paragraphs that introduce an event or problem, or a multiple page document that includes all major details of the case. The document can be given to the learners in its entirety, or, as is more effective, it can be given in segments, sequentially, as they are ready for or request new information. New material can also be presented at each new group meeting. The document can provide all the information the learners need, or the document can be designed to be used in conjunction with other sources of information (e.g., a standardized patient). When preparing a written document, consider organizing the information in the sequence it would present in real life, not reorganized into a formal "case," such as you might present to colleagues. In general, it is best to withhold most of the information initially, or you can defeat a central purpose of PBL: you may deny learners the experience of pursuing their own lines of inquiry and diminish the possibility that they will develop or refine their problem-solving skills.

Clinical materials. A mock-up chart, or segments of a chart, can add a sense of reality to the case, as can radiographic images and other materials that practitioners would have access to when caring for the person depicted in the case. (If the case is based on a real person or a combination of people, you might be able to use copies of real materials, providing that the patient's identity and other confidential information are concealed.)

You as a source of information. You can give learners some initial information (perhaps on paper) and then let learners elicit the remaining information from you. Here you are essentially being an "interactive patient chart," dispassionately revealing information in response to requests, which is different from role-playing the patient, as we discuss next.

You as the patient. Rather than simply giving information to learners, you can play the role of the patient and let the learners interview you.

Preparing yourself to be a patient can be easier than training a standardized patient, but it presents you with an extra responsibility during the instructional session. Also, if the patient you are to role-play is different from you in critical ways (e.g., a different gender, educational level), the role play may seem inauthentic to the learners. You may also find it difficult moving back and forth between being a tutor and being the patient, and the students may have difficulty adapting to your changing roles. If you are coleading the group, one of you can be the patient while the other remains in the tutor role (e.g., introducing the "patient," inviting learners to talk to the "patient," processing the interactions).

Standardized patients/clients. Standardized patients (SPs), sometimes called *simulated patients* or *programmed patients*, are people (sometimes, but not always, actors), who are directed to present with certain problems, symptoms, feelings, and life situations. Scripts for SPs, who are defined as seeking health care in a primary care setting, might include the following:

- pertinent information about who they are (e.g., age, family and work situation, life style, education, cultural and religious heritage)
- the nature and history of their health problem(s)
- what if anything they have done to care for themselves
- other information (e.g., associated health problems, relevant family history)
- where and under what circumstance they will be encountering the learner (e.g., a first visit to a health center)
- their emotional state when they first meet with the learner (e.g., worried, angry)
- guidance on what changes they might go through in response to the various ways they might be approached and related to (e.g., how to respond to sensitive, collaborative care versus impersonal, harsh, or authoritarian care).

SPs can be asked to ad-lib other information in a manner and style consistent with their image of the patient they are portraying, and they can use their own actual medical and personal histories in areas that are not covered in the script. (If people are to be SPs often, it is best to have multiple practice sessions in advance to ensure that they achieve consistency and believability, especially during any ad-libs that may be needed.)

Typically, either the tutor or a student will begin interviewing the SP. When the student who is doing the interviewing or others want to confer about what next steps to take or another matter, a "time out" can be called. This freezes the action during the group's discussion. When the group is ready, a "time in" is called, and the SP resumes his or her role. The same student can continue interviewing the patient, or learners can take turns asking questions. Usually learners just talk with SPs. Sometimes, they also do parts of a physical exam. If SPs are examined, care is needed to ensure that their feelings and dignity are respected.

SPs add a human dimension that isn't possible with paper- or computer-based cases. Students can practice their observation and communication skills. They can focus not only on what information they gather but *how* they gather information. And they can get feedback on how they do. Unlike real patients, SPs can be prepared to handle clumsy questions, awkward or inappropriate examinations; embarrassed or insecure learners; and long, fatiguing sessions. Students can ask whatever questions occur to them. There are clearly many instructional advantages when using SPs. However, recruiting and training SPs takes time. You need to develop a "script" with the key information and provide for rehearsals with constructive critique. For more information on preparing and using SPs, see Barrows (1987).

Real patients.   In a group setting, learners can collectively interview a real patient who has been properly prepared. (Real patients need to know such things as the educational purposes of their participation, how the process works, and what is expected of them.) After students collect information from the patient and summarize aloud what they've learned, the patient can provide feedback regarding the extent to which the learners helped them feel comfortable, heard and understood them accurately, and presented information clearly. After the meeting with the patient, the group can discuss issues that were not appropriate to raise in his presence. They can also talk in more detail about their hypotheses, the mechanisms that might be underlying the patient's problem, and further steps that need to be taken.

Real patients bring credibility and reality to group sessions, and you can give attention to learners' interpersonal skills as they talk with the patients. A potential disadvantage is having to use the patient's real situation rather than being able to program a problem that matches the specific issues that the learners need to address. It also takes time to prepare patients and to later debrief them (discuss their reaction to being in the group, and identify and address any concerns or issues that might have emerged from the experience).

Video triggers or clips. Seeing the people in a paper case (e.g., the patient/client and family members) on a video trigger helps bring the situation to life. Learners can make their own observations and get feedback on their observational skills.

The easiest way to create a trigger is to videotape an encounter with a patient (and family) who you want to feature in a PBL case. (The encounter might be between you and one of your patients.) Then select one or more short video segments from the encounter to use as triggers. If you are seeking very particular footage, you might need to tape encounters with several patients before you get the patient and situation you want. Over time, some teachers build libraries of taped encounters that they can draw on as needed for specific purposes.

You can also get particular footage you want by preparing an actor to be the patient (giving him the kind of information previously suggested for SPs, not a word-for-word script). Then tape him in a real clinical setting (e.g., exam room, hospital room) as he interacts with a real clinician. Select a clinician whose skills and style are appropriate for your instructional goals. Give her a general sense of what you want, but ask her basically to be herself. If you don't get what you want in the first "take" (recording), consider doing a second take. When videotaping, set up the camera to feature the patient so that viewers can easily imagine they are interacting with him. For more information on creating and using video triggers see Westberg and Jason (1994a).

Arranging for other needed resources

When working on challenging cases, students typically need to use a variety of resources. In fact, one of the reasons for using PBL is that it can give students practice in gathering and evaluating information from multiple sources. Some tutors compile lists of resources and resource people from which students can choose. Others want learners to find their resources for themselves. Your choice should be guided by your instructional goals.

What resources are needed or desirable? Think through resource materials that can be useful to the students in addressing the case (e.g., books, journals, monographs, photographs, videotapes, films, laser disks, audiotapes, models, specimens, radiographs, microscopic slides, computerized databases). In addition, identify resource people who could be helpful (e.g., basic or social scientists, clinicians, people in the community).

Do special arrangements need to be made for any of the resources? In general, because of the lasting lessons that can be learned from the process, we recommend having learners do as much research as possible on their own, including identifying and using resources you may not have considered. Nonetheless, you will likely need to make some preparations. For example, you might need to make special arrangements for appropriate specimens, radiographs, and slides to be available. If some resource materials such as books or audiovisuals need to be used by multiple learners, circulation of these materials might need to be restricted (e.g., put on reserve at the library). If you anticipate that learners will want to turn for help to certain resource people, you may need to tell these people what is needed, secure their permission, work out arrangements for their availability, and make plans to avoid excessive demands on their time. Perhaps several students can meet with them at once.

What resources should be available in your meeting room? If the group is meeting only once with no time for the learners to gather information outside the session, you may have to provide needed resources in the meeting room, and you may have to serve as a resource. Even if time is allowed for learners to gather information outside the meeting, having some basic tools (such as a medical dictionary, relevant textbooks, or a model) in the meeting room can be helpful. Ideally, there should also be a computer equipped for searching relevant databases. Think through what furniture and other equipment are needed. For example, students often work around a large table and write their ideas on a surface that can be seen by all of them, such as a chalkboard or flipchart.

Preparing yourself

As you think through the kind of leadership you want to provide, consider the behaviors that Wilkerson and colleagues (1991) found were positively correlated with effective tutoring in problem-based groups at Harvard. For example, they found that effective tutoring was student-, rather than teacher-directed. Tutors trusted students to accurately assess their own learning needs and to determine areas in which discussion should proceed. Once a discussion was under way, these tutors occasionally asked questions to guide the group process or probe for understanding, and they provided some limited information. Mostly, they let the students ask and answer questions, and they encouraged students to listen fully to each other.

The total amount and type of participation by tutors was not as important as the pattern of participation. Whether asking questions or making statements, effective tutors built on the preceding comments made by students. Before intervening, they listened as students developed their ideas through discussions with one another. Also, they tolerated periods of silence that occurred when students had no more to add, while students looked up information in a text, or when group members were thinking.

The students who were in groups with effective tutors selected most of the topics to be discussed, focused on those areas in which they felt the greatest sense of confusion or lack of knowledge, and set an appropriate beginning level of complexity. Their control of the subsequent discussion allowed them to determine the amount of time needed to build a satisfactory understanding of the material.

Ideally leaders of PBL groups are skilled in managing group discussions in the ways just described. They also have a good understanding of the problem solving process as well as some content expertise. Content expertise is needed for designing appropriate problems, for identifying useful learning resources, and for guiding the students' learning. For example, an effective content expert can recognize when learners are caught in a blind alley, are lost in unproductive wallowing, or are beyond their joint capacity for recognizing that they have lost their way. The teacher who is both a content and a process expert knows when and how to use questions to help the learners get back on track. However, tutors with content expertise, without matching facilitation skills, can be tempted to jump in with answers and be heavy handed in directing the students' learning. Thomas (1992) reported that new tutors, feeling the need to share their experience, may dominate up to 80% of the tutorial time. Moust and colleagues (1990) reported that faculty members have trouble keeping their knowledge to themselves, particularly if discussions are in their areas of expertise. Disappointment among some tutors with not being able to share their expertise was reported by Des Marchais and colleagues (1992). Some new tutors at the University of Hawaii tended to revert from facilitators to content experts. This included neglecting an important facilitation task: identifying and confronting student behaviors that interfered with the group's functioning (McDermott & Anderson, 1991).

As we discussed in Chapter 3, Silver and Wilkerson (1991) also found that tutors with content expertise tended to be more directive in tutorials. The authors concluded that content-expert tutors were at risk of endangering the most important goal of PBL: developing students' skills as active, self-directed learners. They suggested that these tutors should go through faculty development activities that alert them to the pitfalls and dangers of their knowledge and authority and habitual ways of functioning.

If you are new to PBL, you will probably need to acquaint yourself with the process and reflect on your role. If you are a content expert, think through how you can best use your expertise to facilitate your students' learning. If you are to be part of a problem-based course, we recommend the following steps: observe effective tutors in action; read about PBL (see, for example, Wilkerson, 1991, a helpful explanation of what it takes to become an effective tutor); discuss what you've read with colleagues; practice being a tutor (e.g., in a simulated group); and invite feedback on your efforts. If faculty development opportunities are not available at your institution, consider attending one of the workshops on PBL offered at other institutions.

FACILITATING PROBLEM-BASED LEARNING GROUPS

In Chapter 4, we presented generic leadership tasks and strategies involved in conducting small group sessions (e.g., creating an environment in which learners can take risks). In Chapter 6, we focused on tasks and strategies involved in facilitating productive discussions and dialogues (e.g., helping learners communicate clearly and consider multiple points of view). Here we build on, expand, and modify some of those tasks and strategies with reference to the specific responsibility of serving as a group facilitator (tutor) in PBL. We offer the following approach as one to consider when reflecting on the approach you have been or will be using. It is certainly not the only approach.

We focus on the situation of helping students learn in the context of understanding and addressing patient cases. However, many of the tasks and strategies we discuss apply as well to working with other kinds of cases and with nonclinical problems and puzzles.

Orienting/Preparing the learners

Early in the session, even while attending to introductions and other preliminaries, we recommend, as usual, that your central task is being diagnostic—finding out who your learners are and what, if any, experiences they've had with PBL and with small groups. The following are some additional initial steps to take.

Ensure learners understand what PBL is and why learning in this way is desirable. If learners are new to PBL, give them a brief overview of what it is (e.g., how the case they will be working on shortly will be the springboard for learning, how they will be responsible for their own learning and will build knowledge together, how you will serve as a facilitator and coach not as a purveyor of knowledge). If the learners are accustomed to subject-based learning, consider talking with them about the differences between subject-based learning and PBL (including the contrasting ways in which learners acquire and organize knowledge) and invite them to explore the advantages and disadvantages of each approach. If learners expect and want you to "teach them" and worry that in the PBL format they won't learn what they need to know, consider inviting them to explore the advantages and disadvantages of the authoritarian model they are accustomed to and the more collaborative PBL model.[9]

Apart from being new to learning in the context of cases or problems, some learners may be unaccustomed to learning through dialogue with others. If that is the case, consider also reviewing with them the general rationale for the discussion/dialogue method of learning presented in Chapter 6.

Take care of big-picture issues. Before turning to the case, consider talking with learners about such matters as how many sessions you will be having together, how many cases you'll be working on, how much time will be given to each case, whether you or other faculty have specific expectations of them, how they will be evaluated, and so on.

Help learners decide how they will work together. In PBL, as we've mentioned, learners often have to make decisions, such as what information they want to gather and what learning issues they want to pursue. To ensure that they make the best decisions, they need to determine ways that everyone's opinion can be voiced and heard (create ground rules that support this), and they need to decide how they will make decisions (e.g., by consensus, by majority rule). If they decide to make decisions by consensus, they also need to decide what to do if time is running out and they haven't yet reached consensus (e.g., revert to majority rule) (see page

---

[9] We present some of the rationale for PBL in the introduction to this chapter. See also Chapter 1. Students may find it helpful to read Donald Woods' book (1994). Although not written specifically for students in the health professions, this book deals with some generic issues in helping students adapt to and gain the most from PBL. You may find it helpful to review that book yourself, as well as his accompanying Instructor's Guide (1995).

43). It's also helpful for learners to establish a mechanism for dealing with disputes (e.g., about the accuracy of information one of them presents) that cannot be resolved during the session. For example, the group might decide that such disputes, as well as other unfinished business, should be recorded on a flipchart so that one or more learners will gather needed information between sessions, and the issues will be readdressed at the next session. (Taking such steps can help prepare learners for being on health teams.) If learners are new to PBL, you might want to postpone a full discussion of how to work together until they have had some initial experience and know what issues they are likely to encounter.

Guiding the learners through the process

Outside of initially presenting the problem, many of the tasks involved in guiding learners through the PBL process are reiterative and overlap. For example, early in each session groups typically generate hypotheses and identify learning issues. They then return to these activities multiple times while progressively building their knowledge and gathering new information. In guiding the learners, the following are some key tasks.

Set the stage and present the case. Before starting the discussion of the case, you may want to present some background information (e.g., let the learners know if the case is based on a real patient story.) Also, since this is an exercise of sorts, learners need to be clear about the goals of the exercise, how they are to approach the case (e.g., are they to find explanations for the information they are given or are they to try solving the problems embedded in the case?): what specifically you will do; and what specifically they are expected to do. In this discussion be sure to include whether they will get all the information at once and, if not, whether you will simply give it to them at a particular time, or they will gather more information themselves. If they are to gather information themselves (e.g., from you or a standardized patient), be sure they know how they're expected to do this. For example, if they will be interviewing an SP, discuss who will interview the SP (e.g., several learners, one at a time) and how the group will move between gathering and discussing information (perhaps using the "time-in/time-out" strategy previously mentioned).

If learners will be gathering information from an SP or from you in the role of patient, before starting the case we encourage you to talk with the learners about the kinds of questions they will ask (e.g., open-ended, closed) and the ways they will ask them, and then pay attention to these issues as they interview you or the SP. Skipping these preparatory steps creates a risk that learners will conclude that such issues are unimportant. They may remain unaware that the kinds of questions they ask and the ways they interact with patients can powerfully influence the quality and completeness of the information they get.

If the learners come from academic traditions in which they were expected to give the "right" answers to teacher's questions and so try to hide their deficiencies, consider taking time to explain that they need to bring the opposite mind-set to this exercise (as well as to the rest of their learning throughout their careers). For example, you might tell them that the intention of the case and session is for them to become aware not only of what they already know but ways in which their current knowledge is insufficient or incomplete. You might also let them know that you will be asking them questions but that your intention is to stimulate their thinking, not to determine if they can give you the "right" answer. You might also discuss how, if they are to become and remain safe practitioners, they need to be continually aware of the limits of their knowledge and set learning goals for themselves.

Help learners identify significant information. When eliciting information from patients, health professionals can be bombarded with a great deal of information and be faced with having to determine what is pertinent and what is not. If patients are not initially helped to be comfortable talking about what they consider to be their most significant problems, clinicians may not learn about those problems until later in the encounter or during a subsequent encounter, if at all.

As learners reflect on the information they've been given or are gathering, help them think about these issues. Consider recommending that group members begin generating on a chalkboard or flipchart a list of what they consider to be the key information, as it emerges. Invite them to edit and add to the list as they continue addressing the case. If appropriate, have them also create a patient problem list, as a practitioner would in a real clinical setting, recognizing that the evolving list will need to change as they refine their sense of what the patients' problems are or appear to be. As your learners become more experienced, consider having them include among the pertinent information the *context* of the patient's situation and problems. The social, economic, and cultural circumstances of the patient's current life can be profoundly important in influencing the onset — and prospects for recovery from — many health problems. Learners need to begin understanding these issues as early as possible.

Help learners begin generating hypotheses. Just as effective practitioners begin formulating hypotheses during the earliest moments of a patient encounter, you can encourage learners to start formulating hypotheses after they've been given or have gathered some initial information. If, for example, the learners have determined that the patient is a 45-year-old man who has had headaches off and on for several weeks, you might ask them to hypothesize about the possible sources of these headaches ("Do you have any ideas, guesses, or theories as to what could be causing the patient's symptoms? What deserves to be explored?").

Learners are likely to generate the most hypotheses if they brainstorm. If you want them to think as broadly and creatively as possible, invite them to call out their ideas and have one of them write on a chalkboard or flipchart. Ask them to defer discussing, rank ordering, judging, or editing the hypotheses until all are listed. Encourage the learners to avoid categorizing their hypotheses (e.g., by affected organ systems, anatomic locations, or physiologic disorders) so as not to inhibit creativity. The lists can be organized later, as the process continues and additional information is gathered (Barrows, 1985).

Encourage the students to add to, drop, and refine their hypotheses as they get new information or reflect further on information they have already gathered. If they fall into the trap of becoming prematurely committed to an early hypothesis, failing to recognize or accept new, disconfirming information, you may need to help them recognize what has happened.

Encourage learners to identify and share what they already know. Questions such as, "Have you had any experience with a situation like this?" can help learners generate hypotheses. You can also help them dig into what they already know, including heretofore unarticulated tacit knowledge, by asking them to share what they know about the various hypotheses they are considering. For example, "What do you know about the links between stress and headache?" "Are any environmental factors associated with headache?" "Do tumors have to be considered?" Help learners bring what they've learned in other cases or courses to bear on this case. ("What have you learned about neuroanatomy that might help you understand why the patient is experiencing pain in this particular way?") As we discussed in Chapter 6, you can meaningfully enhance the value of such sessions by also helping the learners communicate their ideas clearly and listen actively to each other.

***Help learners examine their current knowledge and identify learning issues.*[10]** As we also discussed in Chapter 6, the act of sharing what they know can help learners recognize the extent of and the limits of their knowledge. Also questions, such as the following, which you or others ask of them or they ask of themselves can enable them to realize that their knowledge is incomplete or insufficient. Initially you may need to raise these questions (model what you want them to do), but you can urge them to begin asking such questions of themselves and each other:

- How confident are you about the accuracy of what you're saying?
- Is what you're saying consistent with . . .?
- What is your evidence for making that assertion?

Remember that the *way* you and the learners ask such questions is vitally important. Depending on how questioners phrase what they say and the tones of voice and facial expressions they use, the same words can be felt by learners as friendly invitations to enhance their competence or as unfriendly assaults.

Also, use strategies that encourage learners to speak up when they are puzzled, confused, or uncertain. This includes supporting and even congratulating learners when they identify learning needs. Of course having an evaluation system that rewards rather than punishes them for doing so is essential.

You can help learners make the transition to PBL from conventional learning situations, where they are often discouraged from acknowledging their informational deficits, by emphasizing that the PBL cases are designed to help them bump up against the limits of their knowledge and that identifying their limits is a starting point for meaningful learning. When

---

[10] You can be helped in guiding learners in assessing their knowledge and in setting appropriate learning goals if you are aware of their stages of knowledge integration in your subject area. Norman and colleagues (1989) suggest that novice learners tend to have "dispersed knowledge": list-like knowledge of isolated facts with little conceptual integration. More advanced learners have "elaborated knowledge": the facts and principles of the various areas of medical information are richly organized to support their use in the solution of problems. At the highest level of expertise, knowledge is "compiled" and condensed: clinical cues and contextual information are instantly and automatically recognized. This last level depends on considerable experience and occurs later in or following training. It is possible that the dispersed knowledge of novice learners is, at least in part, an artifact of conventional instruction, in which information is presented didactically, without context or any serious effort at establishing linkages.

the group's collective knowledge is insufficient, pose such questions as, "Might this be an area for which you need to gather more information?" and encourage learners to identify learning issues. To emphasize that you place high value on their being curious, on asking and pursuing questions, and on doing continuous self-assessments, consider, early in the session, asking learners to create a "learning issues" heading on a chalkboard or flipchart under which they list their issues. You can also encourage the learners to each create a personal list of learning issues.

Identify and elicit further information.   If the case is designed to encourage learners to continue gathering information, help them learn to ask themselves, "What else do we need to know?" Encourage them to think critically about the steps they plan to take, asking such questions as:

- Why do we need this information?
- What do we expect to learn from that question (or exam or test)?
- Are there any risks associated with the proposed investigation?

Since a key reason for gathering further information is to test hypotheses, consider inviting learners to reflect on the kinds of information they need for testing the hypotheses they've generated. ("What do you need to know to determine if environmental factors might be a possible cause of this man's headaches?) Caution them to stay open to other possible explanations for the problem at hand. If the learners are interviewing a standardized patient or you, you could use this as an opportunity to reinforce their communication skills by exploring ways to ask questions so as to maximize their chances of getting the information they need.

Summarize, synthesize, and update information, hypotheses, and learning issues.   An important leadership task is periodically summarizing and synthesizing what has been learned and what still needs to be learned. For example, if the group has just gathered more information about the problem, you and they might reflect on such questions as:

- What do we now know about . . . (e.g., the patient and his problem)?
- What appear to be the most important issues?
- How does what we've learned affect our list of hypotheses?
- Do we have any new hypotheses or need to modify existing ones?
- Do we want to relinquish any of our original hypotheses?
- How would we now rank order our hypotheses?
- Do we have any new learning issues to pursue?

As you discuss these questions, have a student make the appropriate additions, corrections, and deletions to the group's lists of facts and observations, hypotheses, and learning issues. Continue helping learners articulate their thoughts clearly, listen carefully to each other, and constructively challenge each other's thinking. During one group session, groups can go through multiple cycles of information gathering (inquiry), hypotheses generation, reflection and analysis, and synthesis.

Decide which learning issues to pursue and how to pursue them. If you and the group will be meeting multiple times to address a particular case, toward the end of each group session, reflect on the list of learning issues using questions like the following:

- What do we need to know to address this problem?
- Are there any learning issues that are not yet on our list that should be?
- Are there any overlapping issues that can be combined?
- Are there any issues that not all of us think are relevant or important?
- Are any of the listed issues intriguing but not directly relevant to our problem?

Particularly if the list of learning issues is long, ask learners to edit and organize the items, eliminating nonessential ones. Then prioritize the remaining items.

If the group is new to PBL or to your institution and community, help them think through where and how they will gather needed information. If learners are not familiar with the resources in your library, consider arranging for a librarian to give them an orientation. Ask the learners to reflect on the kinds of resources to use for the types of information they need. For example, textbooks are not likely to be helpful if the learners need the most current information. If they have not already done so, encourage them to each begin setting up personal information systems. If learners will be consulting with other members of the faculty or with people in the community, help them think through how best to contact and use consultants. In particular, challenge them to think through carefully what they want to learn from the consultant and to formulate specific questions (and how to ask them) before meeting with him or her.

Learners also need to decide which learning issues should be tackled by everyone and which will be assigned to individual group members. As learners divide up the tasks, encourage them to stretch themselves by selecting topics in areas that are new to them or may be difficult for them. If feasible, encourage them to use electronic mail (e-mail) to share hand-outs and visuals they develop or obtain between sessions.

If students come to the session with a mind-set that they do not know very much about health care, consider drawing attention to what they do know. ("Before we end today's session, let's reflect on what you've already brought to this case. Review the hypotheses you have generated and think about the helpful experiences and knowledge you have shared.")

Deal with disagreements.   Earlier we suggested inviting learn-ers to think through how they want to work together (make decisions, deal with disputes). If what they decided to do is not working, you can invite learners to rethink how they can best work together. If, despite reasonable mechanisms for working together, some learners are continually in dispute with each other, be diagnostic. Try to determine if there are other issues (e.g., personal issues) behind these disputes. Also, consider some ways to help the learners manage their disputes (see pages 94–102).

Reflect on the session and plan the next steps and session.   When groups generate lists of hypotheses and learning issues and then review and synthesize these lists, they are summarizing the content aspects of the session. Groups are often strengthened by also reflecting on how they are working together and on identifying ways they can work together even more effectively at subsequent sessions. Before learners leave, they should be clear about what they are expected to do between sessions, what they are expected to do at the next session, and where and when the group will meet again.

Guiding the process at subsequent sessions

Focus on the case.   When groups reconvene, students can be so eager to share what they've learned that they may begin the session by launching into a series of topic-based minilectures. They are at risk of losing sight of the ways in which their newly assembled information needs to be integrated into the larger conceptual framework required for thinking systematically about the problems that provoked their study in the first place. To help keep follow-up sessions from being topic rather than problem oriented, Wilkerson (personal communication, 1995) suggests reintroduc-ing the case at the beginning of each session.

Help learners integrate and apply what they learned between sessions. By beginning with the case, learners will be challenged to apply their new knowledge, rather than just recite it, increasing the likelihood that they will integrate and be able to remember what they learned. After reintroducing the case, have the learners review the lists they created at the prior session, encouraging them to share what they've learned in the context of seeking to understand the case and, as appropriate, updating the lists in light of what they've learned.

As group members share what they've learned,[11] urge them to engage in dialogues rather than monologues, to invite questions, and to check for understanding. When they provide information, consider having them do at least a preliminary critique of their sources of information. (Later you might want them to have a fuller discussion of such issues as the pros and cons of various sources, such as textbooks.) Encourage those who are listening to ask for clarification when they are confused and, if necessary, to constructively challenge what is said. Encourage learners to reflect on the differences between their previous lists and the new lists, including how new information can accelerate and enrich the process of problem-solving. Also notice if acquiring new knowledge and refocusing on the case have led to other learning issues.

Revisit any controversies, disagreements, and other unfinished business from the previous session. Also, invite the learners to reflect on how they've been approaching the case and how they've been working together, and check if there are any changes they want to make before being given or gathering more information.

Introduce more information in the case. Some groups meet multiple times to work on the case they were given or the information gathered in the first session. At each session they go through cycles of presenting and integrating what they've learned and identifying further learning issues, which they then address between sessions. This process can be enlivened, enriched, and expanded by giving the group additional background on the patient. For example, revisit the patient several months after the first encounter at which time new symptoms might have appeared (or the patient might volunteer more information), making it easier to diagnose her condition. Of course, each time more information about the patient is

---

[11] Sometimes a learner will not have done his homework. Well-functioning groups will often let the learner know that they expect all group members to do their fair share.

introduced, learners need to go through the steps described previously (e.g., reviewing and revising their list of significant information and their list of hypotheses, generating more learning issues).

Help learners elaborate on what they are learning.   Since a rich network of connections among ideas facilitates understanding, integration, and recall, encourage students to elaborate on what they're learning, not only by revisiting the case multiple times, but also by explicitly building linkages among the bodies of information they're acquiring. For example, invite learners to apply their knowledge to other situations. ("What if, instead of being 45, the patient was 90? How might that affect what you want to do?")

Toward the end of a sequence of sessions, consider reviewing the patient problem again, inviting the learners to use what they've learned since the beginning to decide if they want to revise their "fact" list and their list of ideas or hypotheses. Also ask them to review and, if appropriate, revise their inquiry strategy, data analysis, problem synthesis, and action steps, including their choices of tests and treatments. This reconsideration and reanalysis can serve both to help consolidate their learning and to refine their skills for future problem solving.

Summarize and reach closure on the case.   Some groups need specific help to avoid lingering endlessly on a problem. They need to learn that total certainty about decisions is not routinely available in the real world of clinical care. Other groups need help to see that they were premature in declaring their arrival at a conclusion. They may need your guidance in recognizing the loose ends and unresolved contradictions that remain.

When the group is ready, invite them to do a final summary of the case. If the problem was based on an actual case, after you and the learners are satisfied that they've reached closure, consider sharing the conclusions of the real case with them. Also ask learners to organize and summarize what they've learned. In addition, if students must take conventional, discipline-based exams, Barrows (1985) suggests helping them organize what they've learned within the relevant disciplines (e.g., by creating lists, taxonomies, and diagrams toward this purpose).

Help learners evaluate their work together.   Encourage learners to critique themselves (e.g., how they functioned as problem solvers, self-directed learners, members of the group). Invite them to comment on each other's self-critique and to offer critiques to each other. And invite them to evaluate how they worked together. Ask the learners to think through what else they want to learn. Provide a critique of their work and your own self-critique. Also consider asking them to give you feedback (e.g., on how you facilitated or interfered with their learning).

Helping learners take responsibility for the group's learning

An overriding task in most PBL groups is helping the learners take increasing responsibility for their learning and for the group sessions. As they assume more responsibility, the tutor's responsibilities change. As we discussed in Chapters 1 and 2, a helpful way to think of our evolving responsibilities during group facilitation can be summarized with the cyclical sequence: diagnosing, modeling, coaching, and fading.

Initially when working with PBL groups, you need to assess where the learners are starting from. Depending on their competence and confidence, you may need to introduce them to (provide models of) ways to approach and deal with problem-solving challenges and ways to work and learn effectively in a group. As learners are ready to begin taking over some leadership tasks, you can shift to serving more as a coach. You then observe and, when needed, provide advice on what they do, inviting them to reflect on and assess their efforts as group members and leaders, giving them feedback and support as needed.[12] As they are ready, you can begin withdrawing (e.g., by being silent, moving your chair out of the circle, even not attending some sessions). However, we recommend remaining diagnostic throughout your contact with the learners and alert to any situations where you need to again be more directive. That is, you need to provide "situational leadership," being responsive to the learners' changing needs.

SUMMARY

The problem- or case-based small group learning format has been making a major contribution in a growing number of programs in the health professions (and in other professions as well). Starting with a case and learning within this context enables learners to acquire and organize knowledge in

---

[12] This support is sometimes referred to in the literature and can be thought of as a scaffold, evoking the image of an adjustable and temporary underpinning that can be removed when it's no longer necessary.

ways that make it more likely that they will be able to retrieve and use this knowledge in real-world situations. The approach to PBL described in this chapter gives students practice in being self-directed learners and in working and learning collaboratively with others.

Leading PBL groups successfully demands a considerable range of skills and understandings. The main tasks of leaders of PBL groups are summarized in the self-checklist in Appendix 7.1. (For a review of the more general tasks involved in leading groups, please see Appendixes 2.1, 3.1, 4.1, and 6.1.)

If you want to be part of an ongoing discussion of PBL issues with educators from all over the world, join the PBL List on the Internet. At this time, the e-mail address for subscribing to that List is: listproc @sparky.uthscsa.edu. In the body of your message, just enter: "Subscribe pblist" followed on the same line by your first and last names (don't use the quotation marks). It doesn't matter what, if anything, you put in the "subject" box.

Appendix 7.1
Planning and Conducting Problem-Based Learning

✔

When preparing for leading problem-based learning groups, did I...

❑ carefully select or design appropriate/relevant/realistic cases to use?

❑ choose cases/problems that were appropriate to the program goals and the learner needs?

❑ choose cases/problems that were both sufficiently focused and "ill-structured"?

❑ formulate the case to include the human dimensions and full context of the problem?

❑ decide how learning issues would be generated?

❑ select or create appropriate resources to use for presenting the case/problem?

❑ do the reading and pursue other preparatory steps?

When orienting/preparing the learners, did I...

❑ gather "diagnostic" information about their prior experiences and expectations?

❑ ensure the learners understood the rationale for PBL, if necessary?

❑ explain the process and our respective roles and responsibilities?

❑ help learners decide how they would work together?

When guiding the learners through the PBL process, did I...

❑ set the stage, explain their and my roles and tasks, and present the case?

Appendix 7.1 (*continued*)

❑   help the learners elicit and identify significant facts and
       generate hypotheses and ideas?

❑   help learners identify, share, and examine their current knowl-
       edge?

❑   help learners identify their learning issues?

❑   help learners identify and elicit further information?

❑   help learners summarize, synthesize, and update information,
       hypotheses, and learning issues?

❑   help the learners decide which learning issues to pursue and
       how?

❑   deal constructively with disagreements?

❑   invite reflection on the session's process and guide planning for
       the next session?

When guiding the process at subsequent sessions, did I...

❑   keep the focus on the case?

❑   help learners integrate and apply what they learned between ses-
       sions?

❑   consider introducing more information about the case (e.g., case
       updates)?

❑   help learners elaborate on what they were learning?

❑   help the learners summarize and reach closure on the case?

❑   help learners evaluate their work together?

❑   throughout all sessions, steadily shift responsibility for the group
       to the learners?

CHAPTER **8**

Teaching Communication Skills

Although communication skills have not traditionally received much attention in many health professions educational programs, there is growing recognition that these skills are fundamental to functioning effectively as a professional and to providing high-quality health care. To some extent, learners can acquire and refine these skills as they work in real clinical settings. However, when they are first learning these capabilities, or enhancing existing ones, or trying to make a major shift in how they communicate with patients and others, they can benefit enormously from also working on these skills in the more protected, more controllable environment of small learning groups.

When learning to elicit sensitive information, to provide instruction and advice, and to exercise other skills that are part of being effective communicators, learners need appropriate levels and types of challenge. When teaching in the unpredictable world of patient care, it is difficult, even impossible, to reliably find and provide the specific challenges that provide optimal learning opportunities for specific groups: easy challenges for beginners, higher level challenges for more advanced learners, and the special challenges needed for learners who need to work on making specific changes in their ways of relating to people.

In groups we can also give learners some of the kinds of practice they need by having them respond to challenges presented in video triggers and by having them role-play with each other or with standardized patients. Knowing that they are not interacting with real patients, learners can feel free to experiment and to take the kinds of risks that can be involved when learning complex skills. They can even develop an appreciation for other perspectives by taking on other roles (e.g., patient/client, colleague). When role-playing or engaging in other exercises, they can pause and request assistance, and they can request custom-designed problems. (Learners can ask that the "patient" act in ways that will give them practice dealing with behaviors they find difficult, such as overt displays of anger.)

Engaging in these activities with only one or two learners at a time can be desirable, particularly if the students have special learning needs. However, pursuing these activities with small groups of students (4–10) can be time and cost effective; it can reduce some duplication of effort, and students can learn from each other. For example, everyone can benefit when learners engage in a role play that is observed by their peers. The role players can get suggestions from their peers, and the observers can learn by reflecting on what was done and on other strategies that might be considered. Learners can take turns enacting the same scenario, enabling them to both witness different styles and learn from seeing the contrasting consequences of various approaches. When jointly responding to video triggers, learners can build their skills by comparing and contrasting their responses with those of their peers. Even when they aren't engaged in specific exercises, group members can work on communicating more clearly (verbally and nonverbally) and on listening actively to each other. If they trust each other, learners can experiment with new ways of interacting (e.g., being more direct and assertive).

Some educators who are asked to lead groups that are to focus on communication have concerns about potential problems, such as students who are uncomfortable role-playing, assessing their communication skills in front of peers, and receiving feedback from others. In this chapter, we discuss leadership tasks and strategies that can help prevent such problems and can make the group experience as effective as possible. To some extent all small groups, even those focusing on topics other than communication skills can provide opportunities for learners to work on their communication skills. The strategies described in this chapter can also be helpful in such groups. In addition, some of the proposed tasks and strategies also apply to teaching other skills in small groups.

PREPARING FOR FACILITATING GROUPS THAT FOCUS ON LEARNING COMMUNICATION SKILLS

See Chapter 2 for a series of questions to ask when preparing for leading groups. See Chapter 3 for suggestions about preparing yourself. The following are additional elements of the process of preparing for such groups.

Deciding on the strategies and resources for the sessions

The following are some options to consider.

Demonstrations.   Learners of new skills need a clear picture of what they are expected to do. Verbal explanations alone are seldom sufficient, unless the skill being introduced is simple or a minor variation on an established skill. In some circumstances, such as when students are beginning to learn a complex skill, it can be vital for learners to witness a demonstration before attempting to perform the skill themselves. In other circumstances (e.g., when refining or adding to a skill), learners often do best when challenged to struggle with doing the task before witnessing a demonstration. Learners can be given demonstrations in a large group before meeting in small groups for practicing these skills. Demonstrations can also be provided in the small groups. When the latter is to be done, or if you feel the demonstration given in the large group needs to be supplemented, consider the following approaches.

Invite learners to observe you in a health care setting.   It might be possible for your students to observe you directly (actually be with you) or indirectly (via a one-way mirror or viewing you on live video) in a clinical setting, where you use the skills they are to develop. This strategy can work for learners who are familiar with the demonstrated skill, but beginners can be overwhelmed, confused about what to focus on and unable to perceive the details of what you do. Also, when learners simply observe you, they have access to only what they see. They don't have access to your *invisible processes*—what you are thinking and feeling while performing the acts they witness.

Show learners a videotape of you using the skill.   Videotaping yourself in a real setting, in advance, using the skills you want to demonstrate in a real setting, and then reviewing the tape with your learners during the small group session offers several advantages. This strategy enables you to capture intimate interactions that might not occur in the presence of others. Also, over time, you can accumulate recordings of events that are not readily available under normal circumstances, such as an interaction with a patient who presents special communication challenges (e.g., a person in a manic state). In addition, you can arrange to tape at your convenience, without having to coordinate your schedule with your students' schedules.

There are additional advantages to presenting demonstrations on videotape. You can stop the playback periodically and talk about your invisible processes, making them accessible. You can talk with learners about what you were thinking and feeling and respond to their questions. You can also replay segments of the interaction, study freeze frames, squelch the audio to focus on nonverbal behaviors, and in general examine the demonstration in ways that are otherwise not possible.

Show videotapes of others demonstrating the skill. Professionally ·produced videotapes are available for learning a wide variety of communication skills. You might also consider videotaping a colleague. As with any videotape, you can study the interaction in-depth, but you don't then have access to the demonstrator's invisible processes, unless the tape provides his or her commentary.

Demonstrate the skills during the group session. Some teachers do demonstrations by role-playing with a student or a standardized patient or by interviewing a real patient. With such live presentations, you can make last minute adaptations linked to the learners' needs. For example, you can invite learners to try using a skill themselves in a role play, and then, if needed, you can do one or more brief demonstration(s), focusing only on what they need help with. If you role-play with students, you are limited by how well they can play their roles. If you work with standardized or real patients, you need to take time before class to prepare them for what will happen. If you work with real patients, you may be limited in what you can do or say in their presence.

Invite a learner to do a demonstration. If one of the learners is already somewhat competent in using the skill that the group is to learn, asking her to do a demonstration can foster collaborative learning. The student doing the demonstration is likely to learn from the process, and if her skill level is only slightly higher than that of the other learners, the demonstration is likely to be more accessible to the learners than would be a more sophisticated demonstration done by an expert.

Tape a classroom demonstration and review it with the group. Another option is videotaping a live demonstration done by you or a student during the group session and then reviewing the tape with the group (offering all the advantages just noted). This approach can be particularly useful when demonstrating a complex task. The learners can benefit from the interruptable review that video makes possible. Recordings are easiest to use when the demonstration is short, so the total process doesn't take too much group time.

Video trigger vignettes. In Chapter 6 we discussed using video trigger vignettes for stimulating discussions/dialogues. Video triggers that present human interactions can also be effective in teaching interpersonal skills. Consider whether it would be helpful to use triggers for any of the following purposes.

Facilitate learners' practice of observational skills. Health professionals need to be astute observers of human behavior. Triggers enable learners to view brief events, describe what they saw, and then re-review the events to check the accuracy of their observations. Prerecorded triggers provide all the technical possibilities previously noted for live recordings: freeze-frames for the detailed study of facial expressions and body language, multiple replays, and squelching of audio.

Help learners recognize and reflect on their feelings. There are two types of triggers that can be used: (1) emotional scenes involving two or more people and (2) scenes in which one person (e.g., a patient) looks directly at the camera and appears to communicate directly with the viewer. (An angry client might say, "Do you realize I've been waiting for you for more than an hour!")

Two ways of using the first kind of trigger are as follows:

- Ask learners to view the trigger (e.g., of a nurse and physician arguing) and then reflect on how the interaction made them feel.
- Prior to showing such a trigger, ask learners to imagine they are one of the people in the trigger and reflect on how this event might feel in that person's shoes. Then ask them to view the tape again, this time imagining that they are the other person.

When using the second (face-on) kind of trigger, invite viewers to adopt a role (e.g., be the health professional who is caring for the person on the video) and be aware of and then verbalize whatever feelings and thoughts emerge in reaction to the person's statement.

Help learners identify their attitudes and values. Watching video triggers of people confronting ethical issues, such as whether to have an abortion or whether to discontinue life support, can help learners reflect on and come to grips with their own attitudes and values. For example, you could show learners a trigger in which an elderly woman in the early stages of Alzheimer's disease asks to be assisted in dying. You could then pose such questions as, "How would you feel if this was your patient?" "How do you feel about assisting people in their dying?" "What do you think of others who do so?"

Help learners rehearse approaches to challenging situations.
Most health professionals are likely to face challenging interpersonal events, such as a patient who is angry because she was kept waiting or a father who needs to be told that his child has just died. Learners can be better prepared for these situations if they've had a chance to view such events in advance and rehearse what they might say and do. You can stop the playback of triggers of such interactions at key decision points (branch points where the interaction could go in a variety of directions, depending on what is done) and say something like, "Imagine you are the clinician here. What would you now say and do?"

This use of video triggers enables learners to share and discuss a variety of strategies for handling difficult situations. In the safety of the classroom or conference room, they can improvise and experiment and then get feedback on their efforts. They can literally rehearse a variety of ways of responding to challenging situations, thus building their repertoire of available options for later use.

Role playing among group members.   Role playing enables learners to practice a variety of approaches in a safe environment. They can be themselves and imagine that they are functioning professionally in a particular circumstance (e.g., talking with a hospitalized patient before he undergoes a surgical procedure; discussing a patient with colleagues). Learners can also take on the roles of others (e.g. patients/clients, other health professionals, administrators, even a clinician who is quite different from them) and have the opportunity to gain some insight into these people's perspectives. Learners can role-play one-on-one interactions (e.g., a learner interacting with a patient), and they can role-play interactions involving more than one person (e.g., a family-counseling session, a health team meeting, a meeting between health professionals and community members).

Group members can simultaneously role-play in subgroups (e.g., they can form pairs and take turns role-playing with each other), or two or more people can role-play while the other group members observe them. Also, subgroups of three or more learners can be formed, assigning one or more in each subgroup to be observers.

Written scenarios (the roles and the circumstances under which the characters are meeting) can be created in advance of the session. Typically, learners who are in the provider role are asked to be themselves and are given instructions that include

- the name(s) of those with whom they will interact and other information that clinicians would typically be given in the situation being simulated

- the circumstances under which this encounter is occurring
- their tasks (e.g., find out why the person is seeking help; convey bad news).

Patients' scripts can include the kinds of information typically given to standardized patients (see page 163). They can be asked to ad-lib information that is not in the script.

Nonactors usually have difficulty portraying people who are significantly different from themselves, so when developing scripts for learners or other nonactors, try making the characters similar to the persons who will do the role playing. To avoid requiring role players to engage in much "make believe," try to develop patient problems that are largely invisible except for facial expressions and gestures (e.g., headache or stomach pain) as opposed to highly visible, difficult-to-simulate problems (e.g., a bad injury; severe shortness of breath). Select simple, common problems that the learners or other nonactors might have had themselves or experienced through friends or family members. Keep scripts as simple as possible. Nonactors find it quite difficult to memorize information and learn lines. Having to try doing so can distract from the value of the role playing. The role plays should be kept brief. In the hands of effective teachers, 5-minute role plays, especially with video, can take 30 minutes or more to review.

As learners become familiar with role-playing and have their own patient care experiences, they can help create written scenarios. During class, you and they can also spontaneously create simple scenarios that don't require written scripts.

The advantages of having learners play the patient roles include the convenience and flexibility of working exclusively with people in the group and the benefits of having the learners experience a little of what it's like to be a patient. The disadvantages are that most learners are limited in their range as role players, and some learners can find it difficult to set aside what they already know about the person who is role-playing the "patient."

Role playing with standardized patients/clients. Learners can role-play with SPs (see Chapter 7), who then provide them with feedback. SPs, particularly those who are actors, can present a wide array of communication challenges. For example, they can be directed to be angry, sad, or seductive, or to have emotional conditions (e.g., depression, anxiety) that can present interpersonal challenges. Learners are likely to perceive SPs as more credible than their classmates. The same SPs can be interviewed by multiple learners, providing the valuable lesson that the same patient can appear to be quite different, depending on the approach and characteristics of the clinician.

However, unless the SPs have been recruited and trained by someone else, you may need to find the time to do so yourself. The steps in preparing SPs include

- creating the scripts for the SPs
- rehearsing them in their roles (perhaps role-playing as if you were a learner)
- helping them understand the kinds of feedback that learners need (e.g., how they, the patient, felt and reacted when learners behaved in particular ways)
- helping them understand the characteristics of helpful feedback
- rehearsing some ways they might provide feedback.

Sharing roles. Typically learners play a role throughout a scenario. Other options include giving "key role players" (learners who are playing major roles, such as the professional who is interviewing the patient) the option of calling "time out" when they encounter difficulty and inviting them to seek help from their peers who are observing the role play or to ask someone else to take over the role. Learners might also role-play a complete scenario and then have others repeat the same scenario. These strategies give more learners opportunities to participate and enable learners to see alternative ways of handling a situation.

Creating and reviewing videotapes of the role-playing.

You can add another dimension to role playing in small groups by videotaping the interaction and then having learners review these tapes in ways we describe shortly. There are a number of arguments for using this strategy. Learners can get potent feedback about their efforts. Those of us who have been videotaped while teaching, caring for patients, or learning a new sport, and then reviewed these recordings with effective teachers or coaches, can attest to the power of such experiences. Without video, teachers and coaches can tell us how we looked and sounded but that seldom approaches the impact of seeing it for ourselves.

Video recordings can help learners identify key decision points in interactions, reflect on the choices they made at these points, reflect on other options available to them and the likely consequences of each. Reviewing recordings can also prompt learners to reflect on their internal processes during role-played events. As Kagan and colleagues have demonstrated (Kagan & Kagan, 1991; Kagan & Krathwohl, 1967), reviewing video recordings of events in which they participate prompts learners to remember what they were thinking and feeling during those events. Recalling these thoughts and feelings allows them and us to reflect on and assess their internal, invisible processes.

Learners can study their facial expressions, body language, and gestures, reflecting on the meaning of these elements of communication and on the effect they might have on patients and others. These nonverbal messages can have a considerable effect on the quality of the care that health professionals provide, yet most learners—and even seasoned professionals—have few occasions in which they get feedback about these behaviors.

Learners can study the recordings further after class. It is often difficult to extract all of the learning potential from a recording during class. If all of the people who appear on a recording consent to the learner borrowing it for out-of-class study (alone, with you, or with a peer), the student may be able to learn even more from the role play experience.

In other words, video, used properly, can help elevate the students' learning of communication skills well beyond the standard we have generally tended to accept.

Written forms for guiding reflection. If there are steps that learners need to take or issues that need their attention (e.g., how to be nonjudgmental) when practicing a skill during a role play, you might want to develop a form that helps them reflect on these steps and issues. (The form might actually be an evaluation form.) You can develop parallel versions of the forms (i.e., forms with the same items but different wording) for completion by you and by the other learners. Learners can use forms immediately after a role play to gather their thoughts before reflecting aloud, or they can fill them out after discussing the role play. Sometimes learners will put reflections on written forms that they don't feel comfortable sharing aloud in the group.

FACILITATING GROUPS THAT FOCUS ON COMMUNICATION SKILLS

Orienting Learners and Being Diagnostic

Use introductions for practicing communication skills.
Even if the learners already know each other, they can engage in an exercise that will simultaneously help them get to know each other better and practice their communication skills. You can ask them to form pairs and elicit from each other something that others in the group are not likely to know (e.g., a student's unusual hobby). Ask each person to first report on what they've heard and then get feedback from the interviewee on how well they were understood and how well their peer conveyed what they were told.

Assess learners' needs.   To help ensure that the session is relevant to the learners' needs and experiences and that they understand and are comfortable with the learning strategies, ask them about their experiences with the skill(s) being developed.

- What experiences, if any, have you had watching others . . .?
- What personal experiences, if any, have you had doing . . .?
- How competent do you feel doing . . .?
- What kind of help do you think you need in developing/enhancing your skills?

Also find out about their experiences and comfort with the learning and evaluation strategies you'll be using (e.g., role-playing, reviewing tapes of their work, critiquing themselves, critiquing each other).

Prepare learners for self-assessment.   If you find that the learners have been in competitive environments where their limitations were used against them, you may have to work hard to help them feel ready and able to be open and candid. Since interpersonal skills are usually closely linked to the learners' self-images, helping them be candid about these skills can be more difficult than helping them be candid about deficits in less personal areas, such as their manual skills or their fund of knowledge.

Ensure that the learners understand that to become and remain competent, they need to be skilled in self-critique. Also, be sure they understand why it's important for them to be candid during group sessions (e.g., if you and their peers are to help them grow, you need to know what they want and need to work on).

When the time comes for learners to critique their work, be sure they know what they are expected to critique. You may need to demonstrate what they are expected to do. If they are to use an evaluation form, ensure that they understand all of the items. Being successful in these activities depends on your skills in creating a genuinely trusting climate in your group. If necessary, review the process of building trusting relationships here (pages 73–75), and more fully in Westberg and Jason (1993).

Prepare learners for giving feedback to each other.

Learners typically are uneasy about giving feedback to and receiving feedback from their peers, particularly if they have mainly been in competitive environments. To deal with this uneasiness, be sure they understand the rationale for peer feedback (e.g., being reflective about their peers' work can help them be more reflective about their own work). Ask learners to discuss what would make it easiest for them to be able to receive feedback from others. Even consider developing some guidelines, such as the following:

- Invite your colleague's self-assessment before providing your feedback.
- Focus on helping your colleague rather than displaying your own insights.
- Before giving feedback, think through how you would feel receiving the comments you are about to offer.
- Use nonjudgmental language.
- Give explicit examples of your observations, being as specific as possible.
- Focus on your colleague's behavior, not on him/her as a person.
- When your feedback is subjective, label it as such ("I feel...").
- Help your colleague turn negative feedback into a constructive challenge.

Demonstrate/illustrate skills.
If you think a demonstration would be helpful to the learners, review and consider the strategies described earlier. Remember to find a way to make your invisible processes accessible.

Providing opportunities for learners to practice

We briefly described two strategies for helping learners practice their inter-personal skills: video triggers (page 186) and role-playing (page 188). Here we discuss some specific ways to use these strategies.

Consider using video triggers.   Triggers are likely to be most effective if, prior to the session, you carefully think through how you want to use them and even some of the specific questions you will ask learners. The following steps can also be helpful:

Set the stage.   Give learners a context (e.g., "You are about to see the first few minutes of an encounter between a patient and practitioner at a health center.")

Present a challenge.   ("Imagine that you are the practitioner. When I stop the tape, tell me what you would say if you were to continue the exchange depicted on the tape.")

Show the trigger. Repeat the challenge. Wait for the learners to respond.

Encourage learners to offer various approaches.   As learners give their responses, be supportive, but withhold both your verbal and non-verbal judgments about their suggestions. Encourage them to practice actually saying what they would say and how they would say it, not just talk about it. For example, if a learner says, "I would try to make him more comfortable," you might ask, "What, specifically, would you say and do to accomplish that?"

Consider role-playing some of the options.   To make the exercise even more real, ask learners to use their proposed approaches in role plays with you or another group member. For example, ask the learner to imagine that you are the patient and have her speak directly to you. You can then respond, and the interaction might go back and forth a few times.

Reflect on the options and their likely outcomes.   Typically there is more than one way to respond effectively to a challenge. Help learners reflect on the approaches they are most comfortable with, and take time to examine the rationale for following or avoiding the various approaches they suggest.

Consider role playing.   Some learners are uncomfortable with role-playing and even resist doing it. The following steps can help learners feel more at ease. Your use of these steps should be influenced by the students' readiness for role-playing, which you can determine in part by asking them about their prior experiences with it.

Introduce the learners to what you and they will be doing. Be sure they understand what they will be doing and why. (We strongly recommend not using role playing initially for evaluation purposes but rather using it to allow learners to freely experiment with various ways of functioning. If appropriate, even introduce some playfulness.)

Address skepticism and uneasiness that might have surfaced when you were being diagnostic. Those learners who resist role-playing often say that it bears no relationship to real life. If any of your learners feel this way or are just uneasy, you might talk with them about how all of us role-play when we first learn new skills or assume new ways of functioning. Until new skills have been integrated as routine parts of our repertoire, we are inescapably playing a role. If we were to avoid all role playing, we would significantly constrain our professional growth.

Invite learners to set up guidelines and ground rules that make them more comfortable. If learners seem worried about revealing their own professional style or limitations in the role that needs to be filled (e.g., a practitioner who is counseling a patient), consider asking them, at least initially, to not be themselves, but to adopt a role (even give them another name and identity). Eventually, as part of maturing professionally, they will need to be helped to confront their own approaches and possible limitations.

Consider starting with less threatening role playing in threes. To ease learners into role playing and at the same time give them a useful experience, consider asking them to create subgroups of three people each: a helpee who presents a problem (one he makes up or that you suggest), a helper who is asked to be an active listener, and an observer. Following 3 to 5 minutes of interaction, the helper is asked to comment on how the process went. Then the observer can describe what she saw, and the helpee can provide feedback (e.g., indicate the extent to which he felt the helper was listening and caring). Then the three students can share what they learned about themselves during the experience. The assignments can then be rotated, so eventually all learners have experienced all roles.

Consider asking some trios to present in front of the group a role play that has been particularly challenging. Emphasize that the purpose is to explore a variety of styles and approaches, not to find "the right answer."

Consider involving the group in planning (other) role plays that will take place in front of the group. As we've discussed, to foster ownership of role playing, learners can help create scenarios and establish guidelines and ground rules. You may also want them to help decide whether students will role-play scenarios nonstop or whether key role players will be able to stop if they get stuck and ask for help from the group. Consider asking the learners to decide how role players should be selected (e.g., by drawing straws, by volunteering). Ask the learners to help you arrange the room for role playing. (Arrange the furniture so the role players will be in appropriate proximity to each other. Make sure that those who aren't role playing can see and hear the exchange.)

Ask learners to set goals for themselves, if appropriate. In some situations it can be helpful for learners to define their goals before role-playing. For example, a learner in the role of health professional might want to practice being more assertive or more focused.

Start beginners with simple role plays. Trying to learn complex skills can overwhelm learners. You can reduce or avoid the discouragement that can accompany excessive challenges by temporarily simplifying their learning tasks (e.g., having learners work on a segment of, rather than an entire, interaction). For example, if you want students to learn strategies for helping patients stop smoking, you could have them role-play only the data-gathering component of the exchange (find out how the patient feels about his smoking and what he's already done, if anything, to stop smoking) rather than asking them to role-play an entire counseling session. Or if students are learning to take a history or do an assessment, you could have them role-play only the first 5 minutes of the interaction.

You can have learners focus on only one of the skills in a multiple-skills interaction. For example, if you want them to learn to be more open-ended when gathering information, you could have them just practice asking open-ended questions. You can simplify the challenge by giving them more time than they would have in real clinical settings and design the roles so that the "patient" has only one problem and is cooperative.

Increase the challenge as learners are ready. You can increase the challenge by having learners move from doing part of an interaction to doing an entire interaction, from practicing a component of a skill to practicing the entire skill, from practicing a single skill to practicing multiple skills at once. You can also provide real-world distractions (e.g., interrupt them with a phone call) or pressure (e.g., tell them that other patients are waiting and they need to hurry up).

Set the stage. Become the equivalent of the director of a play. To help learners get into their roles, provide the context: "Okay, imagine now that . . . ."

Allow learners to get into their roles. Professional actors take time for getting into roles. Consider having a few minutes of silence. Even suggest that learners close their eyes or step out of the room for a few moments, if that will help them take on their roles.

Consider videorecording the role play. For the reasons just cited, you can enhance the value of the experience considerably by making and using a videorecording of the interaction. To get a steady picture, put the video camera on a tripod. To have maximum access to facial expressions, adjust the height of the tripod so that the camera lens is approximately at eye level. If you are videorecording only two people who will stay in the same position throughout the role play, once they are in place you can adjust the camera to get the picture you want and then leave the camera alone; or check it periodically, especially if the participants shift in their seats. If the role play calls for movement or if you have more than two people, then someone will need to operate the camera and follow the action.

Consider having learners take turns operating the camera. That involves them in the session, and it can provide learners who are anxious about role playing with something to do. Regardless of who operates the camera, if you want role players to make their own discoveries as they review the recording, ensure that the camera operator doesn't "edit" while shooting (i.e., draw the viewer's attention to specific events, such as a person's clenched fist, by zooming in on or otherwise emphasizing what's happening).

Helping key role players assess their efforts

The amount of time and detail that can be devoted to learners' self-assessments depends in part on the session format. When there will be only one role play in a session, more time can be devoted to the learner's self-critique than if there are multiple role plays. Also, if learners review videorecordings, their critiques can take much longer because recordings help them remember and consider more than they would otherwise. The following are two additional considerations when helping role players assess their efforts.

Reflect aloud about what they did.   As soon as possible after learners have role-played, invite their reactions and give them a chance to ventilate. Begin with an open-ended, nonjudgmental question. (How did it go? How was that for you?) What they say and how they say it can provide you with information about how to guide the review.

Other suggestions are:

- Review the learner's goals. (Sometimes challenges arise during role plays that cause learners to modify their intended focus or priorities.)
- Before proceeding with a detailed review, invite the learner's overall assessment.
- Be sure the learner identifies both strengths and areas needing work.
- Provide your feedback and invite the other learners' feedback, as appropriate.
- Invite the student to summarize what he has learned.
- Consider giving learners a written form to use, before or after their self-assessment, or suggest that they simply make notes about their reflections, including anything that they are learning that they want to use in the future.

(Initially you can model these steps. As they are ready, group members can join you in accomplishing some of these tasks.)

Review a videorecording of their role play.   When key role players are reviewing a videorecording of their role play, consider inviting them to operate the remote control. Both symbolically and actually, this places them in charge of their review process. We recommend telling key learners that you want them to take the lead but that you and the other learners may signal them to stop the playback at times so you can ask questions or make comments.

There are several ways to review a tape. You can ask learners to focus on one or two themes as they go through the tape (e.g., their nonverbal behavior, the way they asked questions). Or you can ask them to stop at each key decision point. Or you can ask them to stop the tape whenever an event that appears to deserve their attention and reflection (e.g., events that went well and events that didn't go well) occurs. When they stop the tape you can ask them to try to recapture what they were thinking or feeling and/ or to reflect on what they did. If the tape is stopped at decision points you might invite the key role player to reflect on the effectiveness of what she did and what other options were available. Other members might also be invited to reflect on what they might have done. Encourage learners to replay segments and "freeze" pictures so as to study them in-depth.

Helping learners reflect on other roles they play

Invite learners who have taken on other roles, such as patient or other health professional, to reflect aloud on what it was like to be in those roles. Ask them to share their insights and any lessons they want to take away, such as how they want to use what they've learned in the future when relating to patients and others.

Helping learners provide constructive feedback to each other

Learners who role-play can provide helpful feedback to each other, and learners who were observers during role plays can also provide useful feedback. Earlier, we discussed helping learners understand the rationale for peer feedback and jointly developing guidelines for providing feedback helpfully. The following are other steps to consider.

Encourage the key role player to invite feedback from other role players. Help learners understand that they can learn valuable lessons by finding out what the "patients," "nurses," "physicians," or other role players were thinking and feeling, generally and at critical times during the encounter. For example, in talking with a person who role-played a colleague on a health team, a learner might ask such questions as:

- Do you feel that I heard what you were trying to tell me?
- How did your character think I regarded your profession and what you have to offer to the health team?
- How did you feel when I . . .?

Encourage the key role player to invite feedback from learners who served as observers. The learner's questions to observers might include:

- What did you observe about my style of communication?
- Did I seem to be listening attentively?
- What did you notice about . . .?

Invite learners to be diagnostic before offering feedback.
Even if the key role player doesn't invite feedback from others, group members can still offer it. However, caution these other group members to avoid simply blurting out their feedback. Encourage them to first invite the key learner's reflections on the event they want to address (generally by asking a question) and to check if he is ready to hear their feedback.

Intervene if feedback is not constructive.
Even if you have prepared learners for providing feedback in constructive ways, some might still revert to hurtful ways of giving feedback (being sarcastic, putting the learner down). Eventually group members can learn to intervene if such events occur. If they are not ready to do so, you can interrupt. Sometimes, asking the group to pause is enough. Some learners will immediately recognize what they have done and will rephrase or reframe their feedback. Sometimes you might need to help them recognize what's happening with such questions as:

- Do you know why I stopped you?
- How would you describe the way you're giving feedback to Mary?
- How might it feel having someone say that to you?
- What are our ground rules about giving feedback?
- What did we decide are the characteristics of helpful feedback?

Review a videorecording of their role play.
The learners' critiques are likely to be richer if they are done with a video- recording. Group members can ask the key role player to stop the tape when they think there is an issue to explore. They can also ask her to replay certain sections.

Consider asking learners to put their observations in writing.
Writing down their comments can help learners think more carefully about what they observe. An evaluation form can guide their thinking. You can collect their comments at the end of the session and give them to the appropriate key role players.

Providing feedback from other sources

Facilitate feedback from standardized patients/clients.
Some learners may feel uneasy about getting feedback from standardized patients in the presence of you and their peers. To make this process easier and to help ensure they get the information they want and need, invite the learners to ask the following kinds of questions of the "patient":

- Was there anything you wanted to tell me in your role as patient that you didn't get a chance to say?
- What would have helped you feel more comfortable talking with me?
- What if I had . . . instead of doing what I did?
- How did you feel when I . . .?

Standardized patients (particularly those who have been trained to provide feedback) can add their own thoughts directly to the learner or in writing.

Provide your critique. Building on the role players' self-assessments and the learners' critiques of each other, provide your own critique (especially of their self-critiques), modeling the way you want learners to provide feedback to each other.

Using the group experience for developing communication skills

As we've indicated, the entire group session can provide an opportunity for learners to work on their communication skills. Even when they are not engaged in communication exercises, urge learners to work on their skills as they observe, listen, present information, and provide feedback to each other. The following are some additional steps you can take.

Help learners recognize how they interact in the group.
Encourage learners to reflect on how they interact with each other when they are not playing a role. Sometimes it's useful to interrupt the group after an interaction that has potential for helping learners look at their own behavior (provided you are not interfering with an important flow of events). When you interrupt the group (say, when tension is rising), consider asking the involved learner(s) to reflect aloud on what just happened. If they aren't aware of what they were doing, you can (nonjudgmentally) describe what you saw or ask others to do so.

Give learners ways to think about their interpersonal skills. A step that is sometimes needed for helping learners become more reflective about their ways of communicating with others in the group is giving them some ways to think about what they are doing. For example, you can ask them to think if what they do facilitates or blocks communication in the group. You might orient them to this way of thinking by having the group generate lists of behaviors that can facilitate and block

communication. Help them to be aware of behaviors that may grow out of good intentions but have the risk of robbing others of opportunities for growth. For example, well-meaning learners sometimes try rescuing peers who are struggling with a word, issue, or problem. They may try speaking for them. ("John thinks that. . . .") Also, when some members of the group are in conflict, another well-intentioned learner may prematurely try being a peacemaker by, for example, smoothing over and minimizing what's happening. ("Mary doesn't really mean to. . . .")

Help learners identify and practice new ways of relating in the group. As learners recognize behaviors that they are not happy with, they may decide that they want to make some changes. For example, a student who discovers that she frequently interrupts others might want to practice listening without interrupting. A student who is tentative might want to practice being more assertive. When properly facilitated, groups can be safe places for learners to try alternative ways of relating to each other.

Invite feedback from others. Above we discussed learners inviting their peers to give them feedback on their behavior during role playing. Learners can also request feedback on their interactions with others in the group, apart from such exercises. For example, a member could say, "I want to try giving others my full attention while they speak. I'd appreciate feedback on how I'm doing." To help members learn how to ask for feedback, you could model such requests. ("One of my goals as a group leader is to avoid sending nonverbal signals that interfere with anyone's participation. Please give me feedback on how I'm doing.")

Processing and summarizing the session

As we discussed in Chapter 4, leadership tasks include reflecting with learners on what they accomplished as a group and how they worked together. This can also be a time to invite learners to reflect on how they are interacting with others in the group and to get feedback from their peers. Another task is making plans for follow-up. When individual learners summarize what they've learned, you might want to challenge them to set new learning goals for themselves based on what they've accomplished and what they have discovered still needs work.

SUMMARY

Communication skills are fundamental to being an effective health professional. Learning communications skills, as when learning any complex skill, requires specific opportunities and conditions. Small groups, when well managed, can provide learners with some of what they need. In small groups learners can repeatedly engage in safe, systematic, staged, supervised practice of communication skills; be exposed to progressive levels of challenge; witness and critique others; engage in self-assessments of their own practice efforts; and receive constructive feedback on both their self-assessments and their communications practice. As with all groups, those that focus on communications skills need skilled and informed leadership. The key tasks in the effective facilitation of groups that are focused on communication skills are summarized in a self-checklist in Appendix 8.1. (For a review of the more general tasks involved in leading groups, please see Appendixes 2.1, 3.1, 4.1, and 6.1.)

Appendix 8.1
Planning for and Teaching Communications Skills

✔   **Did I...**

Before the Session(s)

❏   review the general steps involved in preparing for leading
          small groups?
❏   take steps, if needed, to remind myself of the perspectives and
          needs of beginners?
❏   select and ensure that I knew how to use any needed resources
          (e.g., video playback unit)?
❏   carefully plan any demonstrations that were done?
❏   select and/or prepare any video trigger tapes that were used?
❏   develop scenarios for intended role plays?
❏   prepare standardized patients, if they were used?

During the Session(s)

❏   use the introductions for the practice of communication skills?
❏   discuss the learning goals, the plans for the session, and our
          respective responsibilities?
❏   assess the learners' needs throughout the session?
❏   prepare the learners for self-assessments?
❏   prepare the learners for giving feedback to each other?
❏   demonstrate/illustrate skills, as appropriate?
❏   provide adequate opportunities for the learners to practice?
❏   use video triggers?
❏   use role plays, including some that the learners help plan?
❏   help the key learners assess their efforts?
❏   guide the learners in providing constructive feedback to each
          other?
❏   intervene, as needed, if the feedback was not constructive?
❏   provide feedback to learners and secure constructive feedback
          from others (e.g., standardized patients), as appropriate?
❏   use the group experience itself for helping learners develop
          communication skills?
❏   engage the group in "processing" and summarizing the
          session(s)?

CHAPTER 9

Processing Patient Care Experiences

Sir William Osler, who shaped much of modern clinical teaching, said that there should be "no teaching without a patient for a text" (Osler, 1903). "Experience is the adult learner's living textbook," Lindeman noted (1929, pp. 9–10). "Experience is the best teacher," advises the well worn aphorism. Patient care experiences are certainly critically important for learners in the health professions, and we recommend starting them as soon as possible, but unexamined experiences are not reliable "textbooks." For learners to dependably extract appropriate lessons from patient care experiences, they need opportunities to reflect, alone and with others (including a skilled teacher), on what they did, what puzzles and confuses them, what they think they are doing well, which skills still need work, what delights them, what angers them, what areas they want to explore further. They need to try linking what they are learning to their current understandings, reflect on the implications of new learning for their future work, and formulate learning goals as well as strategies for achieving those goals. Opportunities to engage in these activities one-on-one with a supervisor are vital, but, for the reasons cited next, engaging in these activities in groups of peers can also be important and enriching.

First, since there is something to be learned from every patient, when peers jointly review their patient care experiences, they multiply their patient exposure and their opportunities for learning. Second, students can learn from the steps their peers took and the consequences of those actions. Third, especially if presenters use a "gradual reveal" approach in presenting their patients to each other, the other learners can have the valuable experience of thinking through what they would have done had they been in the presenter's shoes. Fourth, when learners think through optional ways

of approaching and dealing with situations, they can expand their repertoire of what they can do in future situations, increasing the possibility that
they will be effective. (If learners have only one way of doing things, they
are at risk of approaching all situations in the same way, a possibility that
was colorfully captured by Abraham Maslow in his observation to the
effect that, "If your only tool is a hammer, you tend to treat all problems as
if there were nails.") Fifth, reflection after an action can help learners
develop the vital but difficult skill and habit of doing "reflection-in-action"
(Schön, 1983). This skill is basic for clinicians who regularly need to make
decisions about complex events while they are happening. Sixth, in groups,
students can learn to facilitate each other's learning and develop the valuable skills of peer review. Seventh, group processing can enrich decisions
and enhance the quality of patient care. When learners collectively reflect
on the care of patients, insights can emerge that might not occur to an individual, or even to individual learners with their supervisors. If learners are
from different health professions, the range and richness of perspectives is
likely to be even greater.

Teachers who lead small groups in which learners review (process)
patient care experiences have the usual small group leadership challenges,
such as ensuring that no learner dominates the session and that all learners
are active participants. Additional challenges include finding strategies for
helping learners reflect more thoughtfully on patient care and trying to
balance service obligations and educational objectives, especially in an era
in which many educators are being pressured to devote more time to
service tasks and less to education.

There are many kinds of groups in which patient care experiences are
processed. In this chapter we don't focus on any particular type of group
but deal instead with generic issues, tasks, and strategies. As usual, our
emphasis is on ways to foster learning rather than on the specific *content* of
learning. When reflecting on patient care experiences, it is usually important for learners to include time for reflecting on how these experiences
affect them personally. Although we introduce this subject in this chapter,
we consider it so important that it is the major focus of Chapter 10.

In this chapter we discuss specific tasks facing group facilitators and
suggest resources and strategies for dealing with these tasks. This chapter
is not meant to stand alone. It builds on material presented in earlier
chapters, which is not repeated here.

PREPARING FOR HELPING LEARNERS PROCESS PATIENT CARE EXPERIENCES IN GROUPS

In Chapters 2–4 we present some generic leadership tasks that need to be undertaken as part of preparing for and facilitating groups. Here we focus primarily on tasks and issues that are specific to working with groups in which learners process clinical experiences. Since there are many different kinds of groups and circumstances, some of the tasks and strategies we discuss may not be pertinent to your situation.

Preparing for the session

Clarify or decide who will be in the group. Three key variables in the composition of groups are: (1) the extent of the members' relative similarities in educational levels, (2) their relatively similarities in career goals, and (3) their numbers. If you don't have control over the decisions regarding who will be in your groups, you may be stuck with undesirable situations. Groups that are too heterogeneous or too large can be beyond any teacher's capability. If you can influence your groups' compositions, the following are some relevant considerations.

Up to a point, some heterogeneity can bring richness to the exchanges and can help stretch the participants' perspectives. There is no easy answer to the question "How much group diversity is too much?" As usual, with questions involving people, the answer must begin with, "it depends." In general, even when the learners are all at the same level of education and all in the same discipline (e.g., all third-year nursing students), there are still enough differences among them to create a considerable instructional challenge. If the group is larger than 10 members, it is likely that not all the individual differences among the learners in the group can be adequately accounted for in most group sessions. When groups are made more complex, with learners at meaningfully different educational levels or from multiple disciplines, the range of individual needs can exceed the benefits of diversity.

In hospital work rounds, for example, it's not uncommon for medical students, residents, and fellows to be together. Often, in the press of work responsibilities, these rounds focus mainly on the concerns of the residents and fellows. Although students can pick up something of value from these exchanges, they are often overwhelmed and may feel reluctant to raise questions or issues that they worry will be considered too elementary by the more advanced learners present. Typically, these kinds of rounds are not models of efficient student education or of good learning generally. Some schools, recognizing this issue, hold student-only rounds. In other institutions, rounds are "split." For example, the attending physician might meet alone with medical students for an hour before the rest of the team joins them.[1]

Learners who are from different but related disciples may all learn from each other. Particularly if they are caring for the same patients, their complementary and contrasting perspectives about the care of these patients can help enhance everyone's understandings and improve the quality of care they provide. Further, learning in interdisciplinary groups can help prepare learners for careers in which they will work on interdisciplinary teams or collaborate in other ways with other professionals. However, meeting the needs of diverse individuals is challenging, so care needs to be given to deciding when and how best to do this.

Clarify the circumstances in which you will be conducting the group sessions.   In many schools and programs, the group sessions in which students and residents are to review patient care experiences have two agendas: service and education. In too many situations the educational agenda gets short shrift. If the administrators of your school or program have not set aside sufficient time for both service and education, we recommend trying to help them understand the critical importance of including time for learners to reflect on and learn from their patient care experiences. (See the introduction of this chapter and Chapter 1 for some supportive arguments.)

Clarify the overall learning goals.   All of your planning, including the learning strategies that you and the learners select, should be linked to the session's or sequence's learning goals. So, as an early planning step, you and your learners need to be clear about what the goals are.[2] What do you hope will happen to learners as a result of the session(s)? For example, do you want them to routinely reflect on their patient care experiences in a particular way, with some specific questions that they pose to themselves?

---

[1] See Weinholtz and Edwards (1992) for a discussion of strategies for dealing with rounds that include students at different levels of learning.

[2] Shulman, Wilkerson, and Goldman (1992), suggest that faculty and learners aren't always clear about purposes, process, and content of rounds and can express differing views.

Do you want them to focus broadly or do you want them to focus on a particular area (e.g., whether they elicited the information they needed, how they elicited the information, their relationship with the patient, how they solved problems, the plan and its likely outcomes, the biological mechanisms involved in the patient's problems, the ethical or psychosocial or community implications of the patient's situation)? Are there other people (e.g., a course coordinator) who expect certain outcomes? Will learners be able to help set goals for themselves? Consider putting the major goals in writing if that hasn't already been done. In general, each session should provide overt practice in doing the very things that are meant as intended outcomes. If, for example, one goal is that learners will develop the habit of determining the context of each patient's health problem, that goal should be made explicit (even written down) and strategies should be devised for ensuring that the learners are routinely challenged to engage in that task during discussions of their patients at all group sessions.

Decide when and where to hold the sessions. In general, it's preferable to review experiences as soon as possible after they occur, so they are fresh and accessible. That can be much easier to arrange if the learners are all working in the same clinical setting during the same time. However, as learners are increasingly working alone, in pairs, or in trios at multiple sites in the community, the challenge of getting them together while the experiences are fresh is much more difficult.

Typically patient review sessions are held in clinical settings. If that is the case for you, try finding a quiet space where you and the learners aren't likely to be interrupted, and try arranging for adequate patient coverage (which, of course, is often easier said than done).

Decide on the approach. The learning goals should guide the approach used. However, there may be factors that are (or feel like they are) out of your control. Even if you have to work within certain constraints, you might be able to make some choices. Consider reflecting on the following variables (posed as questions), asking yourself which approaches best serve your group's learning goals.

How many patients should be presented during one session? If you are directly supervising the learners' care of patients, you might need to review all of their patients. However, if you are setting aside protected time for instructional purposes, there are several options. For example, the session could be built around one or two students, each doing an in-depth presentation of one of their patients. Or the session could focus on a theme, and students who have relevant patients could briefly present them. Your decision on these and related questions should be guided by a blend of the learning goals, the available time, and your sense of each learner's needs.

Who should select the patients? You? The learners? You and the learners jointly? In general, the more the learners do for themselves, the more diagnostic information you will get about them, and the more you are likely to help them derive from the experience.

What kinds of patients should be presented? This depends largely on the learning goals. For example, if one of your goals is for learners to understand more about a particular condition, then select patients with that condition. Learners are likely to have the most energy around challenging situations, providing they are not excessively so. For example, in traditional Balint groups,[3] practitioners focus on their "difficult" patients (Brock & Stock, 1990; Scheingold, 1988). In some Balint-style groups, the focus is on difficult relationships (Botelho, McDaniel, & Jones, 1990).

If two or more learners in the group share the care of a patient, how should the presentation be handled? If learners have time beforehand to prepare a presentation, you might ask them to decide how best to do it. If the presentation will be spontaneous and the learners are at different levels in their training, the junior learner should usually start.

How to respond to unexpected problems or opportunities? Particularly if your group session takes place immediately after a patient care session, learners may have encountered unanticipated problems or opportunities that captured their attention. Rather than plowing ahead into the planned presentations, you and the group might decide to take at least some time to deal with these unexpected events. Factors to consider include whether the learners are so distracted that they will have trouble focusing on the original agenda anyway, whether this is an appealing "teachable moment," (a time when students are especially ready for learning), and whether it will be difficult or unfair for those learners who have prepared and are ready to present their patients to now have to delay their presentations.

Should learners be invited to present other kinds of health care challenges? For example, what about problems they are having relating to

---

[3] Groups designed for helping clinicians understand and deal with their relationships with patients, originally created by psychiatrist Michael Balint. (For more on these groups, see Chapter 10.)

other members of the health team? The answer needs to be based on your judgment of the severity of the problems, the extent to which the problems are likely to intrude on the session anyway, and the importance of those experiences that might need to be deferred if time is taken for these unexpected problems.

Should the sessions be unstructured or structured? In an unstructured session students might spend most of their time talking informally about recent patient care experiences. In a structured session there would be more explicit goals and planned activities, probably with more formal presentations of patients. If you have some specific objectives and a limited amount of time, structure is probably necessary. Allowing for some unstructured time offers the advantage of providing access to important issues that you did not, or could not, anticipate in your planning. On the other hand, insufficient structure can bring the risk of having a session in which no worthy goals are achieved.

Should learners be encouraged to do outside reading or seek consultations? Again, your goals, available time, and the educational context should influence your response. In general, both of these activities are important components of continuing professional development throughout clinical careers, so opportunities to practice these skills should be provided.

Should the group meet with the patient (at the bedside or in the meeting room)? Particularly if lessons can be learned from seeing and interacting with the patient, and the patient will be an active participant (spoken with and/or examined, not just talked about in the third person), this can be a valuable part of the group experience.

Decide how learners should present their patients. If students are to present patients, they can do so in traditional ways, or you might want to consider the following alternative approaches.

Presenting patients in narrative prose. You can ask learners to write about patients in ordinary narrative prose instead of in technical clinical language. They can then read the story. Or they can tell the story without writing it. There is evidence that when students and professionals use prose rather than technical jargon, they can uncover knowledge about patients and about themselves that otherwise may remain hidden. In writing, they can gain access to knowledge and feelings that, unarticulated, can remain out of reach. Their choice of language and imagery in describing the patient can help reveal their responses to the patient and their imaginations can supply helpful clinical hypotheses (Hunter et al., 1995). Writing and talking about patients in narrative prose can humanize patients in the learners' eyes, transforming patients from abstractions into real people.

Using videorecordings of the learner's interactions with the patient. Learners can be videotaped while interacting with patients. This is easiest to do when the learner and patient will be relatively stationary (e.g., sitting and talking together) and the room they are in has built-in video equipment. However, the new lightweight video camcorders that function well in low light situations make it possible to videotape learners in a variety of situations.

In Chapter 8 we offered suggestions and several arguments for video-taping and reviewing role-played interactions between learners and standardized patients when teaching interpersonal skills in small groups. The same approaches and rationale apply to videotaping and reviewing interactions between learners and real patients. In brief, learners can do more in- depth reviews because videorecordings give them access to information not otherwise available, recordings prompt learners to remember thoughts and feelings they otherwise tend to forget, and you and the other learners will be able to see the patient yourselves and form your own impressions about the patient and the interaction. Also, associating information with visual images can help learners better remember what they learn (Weinholtz & Edwards, 1992).

Typically, when reviewing a videorecording of a patient encounter, leaners are asked to first set the stage (e.g., talk briefly about any previous experiences they've had with the patient and any goals they had for this encounter). Learners may be asked to do an overall assessment before proceeding with a detailed review. As when reviewing a recording of a role play, instructors can encourage learners to stop the tape anytime they want to reflect aloud about what was happening or what they were thinking or feeling at that moment. If the tape is more than 5 or 10 minutes long, the learner might be asked to select a portion of the tape in advance for review at the group session, or the instructor might help the learner make this decision. We recommend using the ground rule that the instructor and peers can signal the presenter to pause the tape if they want to ask a question or make a comment. (For a detailed discussion of the rationale and techniques of peer review of videorecordings of patient interactions in small group sessions, see Westberg & Jason, 1994a.)

Gradually revealing the patient story/interaction. Regardless of how the patient is presented, students can enhance the learning value of the event by presenting the patient a little at a time (e.g., perhaps mirroring the way the patient presented to them). (If they have a videorecording, they can literally stop the recording at key decision points in the exchange.) Each time they interrupt their presentation, the presenters can invite their peers to talk through what they would do next, before revealing what actually happened. Or they can stop after revealing what they did and see if others have suggestions for optional ways to handle the situation. Either of these strategies can be far more engaging for other learners than merely hearing the uninterrupted recounting of what the presenter did.[4]

Decide on strategies for processing the information presented about patients. There are several possible approaches to organizing the review (processing) of the information presented about each patient. One choice is whether the processing should be interspersed into the presentation or withheld until the case has been presented. A second choice is whether the processing should focus primarily or entirely on the presenter or whether other group members should also be challenged to think through what they might have done and then reflect on the possible consequences of their choices. Focusing on the presenter allows for an in-depth discussion of the presenter's work. Involving the other learners, as we've indicated, reduces their passivity and can help facilitate the presenter's reflections. If you want the other learners to think through what they might have done had they been in the presenter's shoes, it's generally best to interrupt the presentation at key decision points so learners can feel part of the action, rather than trying to make decisions in retrospect. If all group members are to decide what they would do in a given situation, a third choice is whether to have everyone commit themselves before reflecting on the implications of each decision or whether first to reflect on what the presenter did, and then have the others indicate what they would do, and process what they say. A fourth decision involves deciding what to focus on. Some sample possibilities are (a) problems and issues that the presenter has identified, (b) the steps that the presenter engaged in when interacting with the patient, (c) the learner's relationship with the patient.

The focus can be on one or on multiple topics. If you are reviewing a

---

[4] This form of "iterative hypothesis testing" is becoming recognized and more widely used in medical writing, as in the clinical problem-solving series that are now regular features in the *New England Journal of Medicine* and the *Journal of the American Medical Association*.

videotape of the interaction, you can track some of these issues over the duration of the encounter and dwell more specifically and easily on relationship and communication issues and on steps in problem solving. If the presenter will be meeting again with the patient, attention needs to be given to next steps and follow-up.

Clearly, the list of choices and options can be substantial, and we haven't listed all the possibilities. Effective leadership involves thinking through all available options and selecting which will likely work best in each unique instructional situation.

Make necessary advance arrangements.   Ensure that a suitable room is available and that the learners or others will bring patient charts, radiologic studies, or other materials needed when discussing their patients. Be sure that a chalkboard or flipchart is available so that written reinforcement and summaries of key points can be provided. If learners are to be videotaped, arrange for that to be done and for playback equipment to be available in the meeting room. Ensure that informed consents have been obtained from patients and colleagues, as appropriate.

FACILITATING THE GROUP SESSION

Orienting learners

Students almost always need some transition time for moving from their previous activity to the group activity. This is particularly true when they have just been caring for patients. Allowing students a few minutes to interact informally (e.g., in twos or threes, or as a full group, especially if it is relatively small) before getting under way can also provide you with diagnostic information about the learners' current states of mind and concerns. See pages 73–82 for a review of initial leadership tasks and strategies. Be sure there are ground rules that protect the patient's privacy, both inside the group and in conversations with others outside the group. If the learners have been accustomed to rounds or other groups that were primarily competitive, and you want to use a collaborative approach, you may need to help them understand why collaborative learning is preferable, and you may need to show them how to function in collaborative ways.

Leadership tasks at the beginning of subsequent sessions include reviewing the agenda that was planned for the day, finding out if there have been any events (e.g., new patient challenges) that cause the learners to want to revise the agenda, and making whatever changes are needed in the agenda.

Helping learners present their patients/clients clearly

Group sessions that are built around learners' presentations of patients can be suboptimal if learners don't present their patients clearly, in interesting ways. The following strategies can help learners present in clear and engaging ways— a skill they can use throughout their careers.

Encourage learners to think about their goals. Invite learners to think about what they would like to get out of their presentations and the reviews of their patients (e.g., some ideas about how to deal with challenging relationships, a better understanding of a complex health problem). Also, encourage them to think about what they'd like their peers to get out of their presentations and reviews.

Be sure that learners are clear about the kinds of information they need to present. In some institutions, students complain that each faculty member wants a different kind of presentation and that students squander time trying to figure out what each teacher wants. You and the learners should think through carefully what information needs to be included in a presentation (including visuals), in what sequence, so that all of you can be maximally helpful to the presenter and each other. You might even write the format for the presentation on a flipchart or chalkboard or put it in a handout. If you are in an institution where an effective presentation format is regularly used, you may choose to help students learn that format. (You might make that an explicit learning goal.)

Develop/use visuals that can enhance presentations. To help listeners grasp the key details of their cases, presenters can put symptoms, findings, and problems on a flipchart, chalkboard, or handout. Presenters can gradually reveal this written information or provide it all at once. Visuals can help make patients and their problems come to life and be more thoroughly grasped. Presenters can show pictures or slides, make drawings of physical findings or anatomical structures, and show radiological images. A genogram can help give listeners a picture of patients in the context of their families. Such visual aids are particularly helpful to learners who cannot easily grasp information presented only verbally.

***Agree upon whether, when, and how to interrupt presenta-
tions.***   If you choose to have students do somewhat formal presentations followed by processing, instead of mixing the two, you and they need
to decide whether and how to interrupt the presenter. Weinholtz (1983)
suggests that you need to consider the frequency of the interruptions and
the type of questions you ask: whether for clarification (e.g., "How did he
describe his pain?") or for "probing" ("What does hepatomegaly mean to
you?").

We suggest that you try making all presentations as interactive as possible, but doing so, as we have described, requires that the learners be given
adequate preparation. Before the first student presents, you might develop
some guidelines. For example, the group might decide to limit questions to
those that seek clarification, unless presenters indicate they are comfortable with more probing interruptions. Then again, for the reasons cited
earlier, the sessions might be most helpful if presentations follow the
"gradual reveal" approach with questions inserted as needed. In general,
we recommend developing a consistent style so that learners come to know
what to expect and can prepare themselves appropriately. By creating a
noncompetitive climate, you can help the learners be more focused on learning and less on making a good impression so they are less bothered by—
and may even welcome—interruptions.

Facilitating the learners' reflection and self-critique

As we discussed in earlier chapters, an overriding leadership task is creating a safe environment in which learners can be candid about the questions
and concerns that emerge from their work. If learners are unfamiliar with
self-critique, you may need to help them understand the rationale for doing
it, and you may need to help them understand when and how they are
expected to critique their work. For example, after presenting a case, you
might want learners to spend a few minutes summarizing what they thought
went well and what didn't, what they learned, and what questions they want
to pursue. The following are some additional tasks when helping learners
engage in self-critique.

***Identify goals (and criteria) against which to examine per-
formance.***   If possible, prior to interacting with the patient they are to
present, learners should be clear about their goals for the encounter (e.g.,
eliciting a complete family history). These can be goals the learners set for

themselves or goals formulated by you or others. As learners begin reviewing the encounter, they can reiterate the goals as reminders of what they were trying to achieve.

Identify questions learners can ask themselves. Learners, particularly beginners, can become overwhelmed by the task of reflecting on their care of patients. Goals can help learners focus, as can questions that embody the goals. Some sample questions: "What did I learn about the patient's views of her condition?" "What did I learn about why the patient sought help at that particular time?" If learners are reviewing a videorecording of a patient interaction, there are questions they can ask themselves every time they stop the tape, such as, "What options was I considering at that moment?" Since it is important for learners to be routinely reflective while caring for patients, some of the questions they ask at review sessions might be questions you encourage them to ask themselves during or following all patient encounters.

Ask questions that help learners reflect more deeply. After the learners' initial reflections and self-assessments, help them reflect on issues that they didn't include, if any. ("What about . . .?" "Did you give any thought to. . .?") If you think a learner didn't delve deeply enough into some areas, encourage him to go further. ("You've identified two plausible explanations for that finding. Can you think of any others?") If a learner is reviewing a videotape and passes over an important event, consider stopping the tape and asking if she noticed anything she'd like to comment on. If she's still unaware of any issues, ask her to watch the segment again, perhaps with a prompt from you. ("As you review that segment, notice what the patient was doing while talking about his pain.") The more you help learners make their own discoveries, the more they are likely to learn.

Invite the presenter to consider options. There is often more than one effective way to approach a situation, and it is important for learners to develop a repertoire of choices for actions they can take in various situations. So, even if what the presenter did at a given decision point was effective, invite him to consider other options, including the possible consequences of each of these options. If the focus is on interpersonal issues, encourage the learner to role-play one or more options, instead of just talking about them. ("Donna, instead of telling us what you might have done, why don't you show us how you might handle this situation. We need a volunteer to be Donna's patient.")

Facilitating the involvement of all the learners

As we discuss next, all learners can be asked to help facilitate the presenter's reflections and self-critique. In addition, you can invite the other learners to do the following:

Invite learners to consider what they would have done and to propose options. We have suggested that the presenter could gradually reveal the patient's story, stopping at decision points to let the other learners decide what they would have done. If you do not want the learners to influence each other's decisions, you can ask them to make a note of what they would have done before having them share their thoughts aloud.

To reduce the risk that the presenter will feel threatened by the presentation of other options, ensure that all learners understand that they can be most effective if they have a rich repertoire of optional strategies and that considering each other's suggestions is a way to build that repertoire. When other leaners have options to suggest that deal with interpersonal issues, consider asking them to role-play what they would do.

Invite presenters to seek their peers' input. In conventional presentations, learners might turn to their teacher with questions. Instead, encourage them to turn to each other and to pull together the group's knowledge. As in problem-based learning, when the group's knowledge is insufficient, members can identify their learning issues and jointly decide how they will pursue those issues. If there are pressing patient care issues to be dealt with on the spot, you might serve as a resource. As we discuss shortly, all learners can participate in elaborating on the case.

Ensuring that learners provide feedback constructively

As we've discussed, if learners are not accustomed to giving each other feedback, you might need to help them understand why doing so is important and help them learn ways to provide feedback constructively. The following are two additional steps.

Invite presenters to indicate what they hope their peers will provide. If learners are to grow professionally, they need to know how to seek help from each other. Presenters can be encouraged to practice asking for help by routinely letting their peers know what they need and want. For example, before reviewing a tape, a student might say something like, "As you know, I've been trying to get patients more involved in their own care. Please give me feedback on how you think I did with this patient."

Help learners ask questions that will help their peers be more reflective. If there are some kinds of questions that you'd like the learners to ask each other regularly (e.g., "How confident are you that the patient understood your explanations?"), you can identify these questions, provide a model of how to ask them, and even have the learners write them down and practice using them.

Helping learners build and elaborate their understandings

To help learners build knowledge, encourage them to anchor what they are learning to what they already know. For example, you might say, "Does this patient's condition remind you of anything you've encountered before?" If it does, you can help learners explore the similarities and the differences. If students are having trouble understanding a concept, you can help them reflect on what they already know and build on that.

Students are most likely to be able to link their new learning to their current knowledge and apply it to future situations if they identify underlying principles, concepts, and strategies. For example, after learners have explored the details of a particular case, you might invite them to step back and try identifying the biological principles that explain this patient's shortness of breath, or you can use a reverse strategy. For example, if learners have been studying a biological, psychological, or family systems model, you can ask them to try exploring ways that model applies to the patient they are discussing. (In Chapter 7 we discussed how cases designed by faculty members can serve as the launch pad for PBL. So too the real cases presented by learners can serve as springboards for exploring a variety of biological, psychosocial, and ethical issues.)

To help students further elaborate on their understandings, consider giving them brief hypothetical situations that they might encounter in the future. Ask them how they would apply what they are now learning to those future situations.

Helping learners summarize what they learned and make follow-up plans

In previous chapters we've discussed how learners are likely to get the most out of sessions if they take time to pull together what they've learned and identify what they want to explore and work on further. In patient review sessions, we recommend inviting the learners who have presented cases to begin this process. Others can then also summarize what they've learned and what they want to pursue further. If the group has been making a list of learning issues, this list can be reviewed. If appropriate, learners can volunteer to research various topics and report back. Also, important lessons from patient care are often lost because many practices lack adequate mechanisms for tracking the process and outcomes of care. Consider finding ways to help learners do follow-ups with their patients so they can be aware of the progression of their patients' conditions and the impact on the patients' well-being of actions taken by them, the patient, and others.

Encourage learners to reflect on how the group worked together, both what went well and what they'd like to change for future meetings. Be sure they know what they need to do in preparation for the next session and when and where the group will next meet.

In the thick of daily pressures it can seem distracting and burdensome to try finding time for these wrap-up activities. Yet, without consolidating and process-enhancing activities, learners may derive less from each session than they might have, and unnecessary activities and inefficient approaches can persist from session to session. Ultimately, more time is usually wasted by skipping these steps than would have been needed for including them as part of the process in the first place.

SUMMARY

If learners are to derive the maximum benefit from their experiences they need opportunities to pause and reflect on those experiences. Although learners need to do some of this "processing" with individual supervisors, one-on-one, having the additional opportunity for reflecting aloud with peers can provide many added benefits. In the self-checklist in Appendix 9.1 we summarize the main tasks involved in preparing for and leading small groups that focus on reviewing learners' patient care experiences. (For a review of the more general tasks involved in leading groups, please see Appendixes 2.1, 3.1, 4.1, and 6.1.)

Appendix 9.1
Preparing for and Processing Patient Care Experiences

✔

Before the (first) session, did I...

☐ clarify or decide who and how many would be in the group?

☐ clarify the circumstances in which I would be conducting the group sessions (e.g., service vs. education focus)?

☐ clarify the overall learning goals and decide when and where to hold the session(s)?

☐ decide on the approach we would use (e.g., how many patients, who would select them)?

☐ decide how learners should present their patients?

☐ decide on strategies for processing the information presented about patients?

☐ make all necessary advance arrangements for learner preparation resource materials, etc.?

During the session(s), did I...

☐ provide appropriate/adequate orientation for the learners?

> help the learners present their patients/clients clearly and interestingly

☐ ...encourage learners to think about their goals?

☐ ...ensure that the learners were clear about the kinds of information they needed to present?

☐ ...encourage learners to develop and use visuals that could help enhance their presentations?

☐ ...decide with the learners whether and when to interrupt the presentations?

Appendix 9.1 (*continued*)

>   facilitate the learners' reflection and self-critique?

❑   ....help the learners identify goals and criteria against which to examine their performance?

❑   ....identify questions the learners could ask themselves?

❑   ....ask questions that helped the learners reflect more deeply?

❑   ....invite the presenters to consider options to the approaches they used?

>   facilitate the involvement of all the learners

❑   ....invite the other learners to consider options to what the presenter did?

❑   ....invite the presenters to seek input from their peers?

❑   ....ensure that the learners provided feedback to each other constructively?

❑   ....help learners build and elaborate their understandings?

❑   ....help the learners summarize what they learned and make follow-up plans?

CHAPTER 10

Providing Support and Fostering Personal Growth

Emotional and social maturity are needed by health professionals, if they are to provide sensitive, high-quality health care. In face-to-face encounters, health professionals are themselves key instruments of the care they provide. They can be as potent as a strong medication, with similar possibilities for inducing positive results or negative side effects (Balint, 1957). The extent to which health professionals can detect and address emotional clues from patients and be supportive and empathic depends in part on their awareness of and comfort with their own feelings, values, and personal issues. The ways that health professionals function as people and their ways of relating to patients can profoundly influence what patients reveal to them about themselves and their conditions, the extent to which patients feel free to ask questions and be candid about their concerns, the value and credibility patients attach to the information and advice the professionals give them, and more. Personal maturity is also needed for navigating successfully through educational programs, for having a stable personal and professional life, and for being a healthy person.

Helping learners be or become optimally mature, self-aware, emotionally strong health professionals who are comfortable with their feelings is (or should be) a central part of our instructional responsibilities. We and our programs have been less than fully successful if we have not helped prepare them for providing sensitive, compassionate, whole person health care.

Becoming a health professional can be a life-changing process. Learners not only have to face the usual pressures of higher education (e.g., passing examinations, dealing with difficult instructors, trying to cover the costs of their education), they also need to engage in many stressful acts, including some that people are normally discouraged or prohibited from experiencing (e.g., asking highly personal questions of near strangers, touching strangers in intimate places, probing and cutting into people's bodies). Learners in the health professions need to be with people at some of the most emotionally demanding times of their patients' lives—births, grave illnesses, death. Some of the interventions they undertake (e.g., medications they give, procedures they do) can cause pain and can even put people's lives at risk. And they face moral challenges.

When learners are unprepared for dealing with the many powerful experiences encountered in becoming a health professional and providing health care, and when learners don't have opportunities during their professional education to "process" these experiences, they can resort to adaptive mechanisms that may be hurtful to themselves and others. When learners don't have a safe place in which to express their anger, sadness, anxiety, or despair, they are more likely to resort to potentially hurtful adaptive strategies: blocking their awareness of their own feelings toward patients in an effort to avoid getting hurt, using alcohol or drugs to dull their pain, blaming others because it is too painful to take responsibility for their own actions, and lashing out at vulnerable people, including patients and subordinates, because they can't contain or don't understand their feelings. They can become less rather than more caring and compassionate.

Effective small groups can help offset some of the negative influences of health professions education by providing learners with a place where they can have a safe emotional outlet. Just being able to talk about what it felt like to dissect a human body, to see people in great pain, to watch a child die, or to be publicly rebuked for doing a procedure in a disapproved manner can give learners a sense of relief and make it more likely that they will be able to make constructive progress in their personal development (Hahn et al., 1991). Being able to reflect on these experiences with a skilled facilitator and peers increases the likelihood that these experiences will serve as stimuli for growth rather than only as debilitating events. In groups, learners can also explore the sources of some of their stress (e.g., ethical quandaries) and learn strategies for dealing with highly charged situations in ways that can help them throughout their careers. Further, if learners are feeling anxious about an upcoming event, such as a difficult new rotation, the group can help them prepare.

In small groups, learners can discover that they aren't the only ones experiencing emotional isolation. Particularly in some fields in the health professions, students do not have opportunities within their traditional curricula to talk openly about their feelings. Coombs and colleagues (1990) reported that the emotional isolation felt by many medical students and resident physicians is reinforced by classmates who project the defensive facade of calm, self-assured achievement, a mask of "relaxed brilliance." In male-dominated settings, "emotional composure often bordering on machismo is valued." Openly expressing one's feelings among peers brings the risk of being labeled as "soft" or "weak."

Students in supportive groups may be more willing to take the emotional risks involved in some meaningful learning. Some students and health professionals try protecting themselves from embarrassment and pain by avoiding situations in which they might feel vulnerable or by putting up walls when they are unavoidably in such situations. For example, learners and practitioners who don't think they can handle a patient's display of sadness sometimes use nonconstructive strategies, such as changing the subject, to keep from having to be in the presence of a crying patient. Learners and practitioners who are not comfortable with dying and death avoid visits with dying patients. Learners who try protecting themselves in these ways may indeed spare themselves some pain, but they are also likely to miss rich opportunities for personal growth and for being helpful to others. If learners know that they don't have to be alone in handling such situations, that they have the support and understanding of their leader and group members, some may take emotional risks that can lead to meaningful learning and prepare them for being far more effective in their careers and lives.

As the high levels of divorce, substance abuse, depression, burnout, and other negative consequences of stress among health professionals attest, studying and providing health care can be highly stressful (Coombs et al., 1990; Kleehammer, 1990; Marchard et al., 1985; McKegney, 1989; Sheehan et al., 1990). Learning to deal with the stresses of health care during their basic professional education is likely to prepare learners to handle such stress more effectively as professionals. In addition, positive experience with providing support to each other in small groups can lead learners, as professionals, to seek out or form support systems with colleagues. By having colleagues who are mutually supportive, to whom they can turn for guidance and from whom they get friendly challenges when needed, they are likely to be helped to remain healthy throughout their careers. Also, if learners develop a capacity for providing constructive feedback and other educational skills, they are likely to have much to contribute to colleagues.

In some institutions, learners are given opportunities to explore the personal, human dimensions of becoming health professionals, individually and in groups. In a few programs students belong to support groups that meet regularly for one or more years. In too many programs, though, learning is focused almost exclusively on cognitive and technical issues. Little or no attention is given to the learners' personal reactions to the experiences they are having—to their feelings and values. Teachers who want to include these issues in the curriculum are given little encouragement and may be actively discouraged from doing so.

Readers who are sympathetic to the need for a focus on these human issues, but who are faced with skeptical colleagues, might consider presenting their colleagues with the arguments just offered and some of the rationale for fostering learning in small groups presented in Chapter 1.

In the remainder of this chapter we explore tasks and strategies that can help educators who conduct groups devoted to issues of personal growth (or who want to include some personal growth issues in groups devoted primarily to other topics) be facilitators of helpful experiences for their learners.[1]

PREPARING FOR THE INITIAL GROUP SESSIONS

In Chapters 2 and 3 we present some generic tasks and strategies that can help leaders prevent unwanted surprises and be prepared maximally for working with their groups. Here we revisit a few of these tasks, focusing on issues pertinent to leading groups that deal in part or largely with personal issues. Such groups can take many forms, so some of the following tasks might be more pertinent than others for groups you conduct.

Making general preparations

In addition to considering the issues raised in Chapter 2, we recommend also reflecting on the following questions.

To what extent is the learners' personal growth valued at your institution?   The extent to which psychosocial growth is valued at your institution is likely to have an impact, at least initially, on your group sessions. If, for example, learners' feelings and values are generally disregarded, or even devalued, you will likely need to bring extra effort to the task of preparing learners for talking about these aspects of their lives. Be

---

[1] We deal primarily with issues of self-awareness and emotional maturity. We do not deal with the important related component of professional maturity: moral development. For an overview of current research and thinking in this area, as applied to the health professions, see Rest and Narváez (1994).

prepared for the possibility that some students, having adopted the mind-set of some of their role models, or having taken on protective strategies, may initially seem overtly disdainful of your efforts. You will need to be patient with them and yourself while helping them make the transition to a different, more open, way of functioning.

Is the group part of a required course at which attendance is expected? If it is, there may be learners who will come to the sessions only because of this requirement. If you suspect that you might have group members who don't want to be there, before the first session try to learn what you can about their concerns. Depending on the goals for the group, you (and your colleagues) might want to make the sessions elective so that only students who feel ready for such groups attend them. On the other hand, if you (and your colleagues) decide that these sessions are vital, not optional, components of the curriculum, you may need to provide some individual counseling to help the most resistant (or frightened) learners gain some understanding and comfort with groups that have a personal focus. If you are uncertain whether such groups belong in the core curriculum of your program, we invite you to consider the possibility that these issues are actually more basic and necessary for professional development than some of the subject matter content of some conventionally required courses.

Will the learners be evaluated and if so on what criteria? Learners are likely to do what they think it takes to get a positive evaluation, so ensure that if you must formally evaluate them, these evaluations won't get in the way of their comfort or openness. For example, learners are more likely to be comfortable with evaluation efforts that focus on the extent to which they make an effort to participate in the process, as opposed to what they say or how much they reveal. Also be sure that you aren't expected to do anything that makes you or the learners uncomfortable (e.g., share with administrators information that learners provide in confidence). To help encourage openness in groups that include or focus primarily on issues of personal growth, some programs do not formally evaluate the learners' participation or work in such groups. If you are based in a grade-oriented, competitive institution, there is the risk that some of your learners will devalue such groups since they may have been influenced by the local culture to give their full attention only to those activities that are "rewarded" with grades.

Deciding on an approach

The following are some of the more common approaches to organizing support-oriented small groups.

Unstructured, open ended. In an unstructured, open-ended group there typically is no agenda other than the general intention of helping learners examine their experiences and recognize and explore their concerns and issues. If multiple issues are identified, the group might prioritize them, deciding which to deal with at the current session and which to address later.

Theme focused. Some groups (or faculty) pick one or more themes in advance of the discussion. Learners talk about their own experiences that are relevant to the theme. A theme-focused group often begins with some form of "stage setting." For example, someone might briefly articulate an issue, such as how to remain kind and supportive to patients who engage in behavior you personally abhor or how to balance the demands of school with the obligation and desire to be with family and friends. Or the group might begin with the reading of a provocative poem or article related to the theme. Or a question can help start the discussion: "How did you feel when you took care of your first patient?" "What were your thoughts and feelings as you sacrificed animals in the research lab?" "Have you ever witnessed a student cheating on a test? How did that make you feel?" "What is it like for you to take care of patients who are dying?" If you anticipate that learners will be uneasy talking about feelings and values, you can start with somewhat safe, noncontroversial issues and gradually move toward tougher issues.

Event focused. If learners are at the same level, in the same program, and are having similar experiences, the sessions might focus on upcoming events that learners are anxious about or past events that engendered strong feelings.

Patient or relationship focused. In the previous chapter we discussed several ways learners can present patients (e.g., in a traditional case presentation model; in story form). We recommend routinely encouraging learners to reflect on their relationships with their patients regardless of the presentation style used in your group.

Balint Groups (and their variants). In the 1950s, Michael and

Enid Balint (Balint, 1957) introduced seminars for helping general practitioners study their relationships with patients. Although currently this model is used primarily by medical residents, physicians, and medical students, the model and its variants can be used by other health professionals. Seminars typically begin with an unscripted case presentation by one of the group members. As the speaker presents the case, the leader and group members try to keep the discussion focused on the presenter's feelings. They also draw the presenter's attention to the group process when it appears to parallel the doctor–patient relationship (e.g., when the way the presenter relates to one or more group members seems similar to the way he relates to the patient being discussed). Intragroup dynamics that impact the sessions (e.g., domination of the process by a group member) are also discussed.

Botelho and colleagues (1990) report that in traditional Balint groups there is a single leader who uses an authoritative style within a psychodynamic orientation. The subject is a difficult patient and the initial focus is the doctor–patient relationship. In Balint-style groups that use a family systems approach, there are coleaders whose style is facilitative. The subject is any difficult professional relationship and the initial focus is on family issues.

Inviting learners to keep journals and read autobiographical accounts

Journals in which learners record significant experiences and their personal reactions to these experiences can be a source of themes for group sessions. The act of journaling can help learners become aware of sources of pain and joy in their lives. Also, writing about their personal reactions to powerful events can itself be constructively cathartic and therapeutic. Reading autobiographical accounts by learners in the health professions, health professionals, and patients can help learners identify issues that are important to them and can stretch them by providing exposure to new experiences and reflections.

Preparing yourself

Just as it is difficult to help patients deal with feelings and events if we are unable to deal with them ourselves, so too is it difficult to help learners with their personal responses to becoming health professionals and taking care of people if we haven't come to terms with such issues ourselves. If you are a health professional, consider reflecting on some of your most moving experiences as a student, how you dealt with those experiences, what you learned from them. Also, reflect on your current experiences and issues.

If learners are not accustomed to talking about feelings in groups and if some have problems doing so, you may initially need to be fairly active, modeling the ways you want them to be helpful to each other and facilitating their self-discoveries. However, remember that if leaders become too directive—in effect, taking over the group—participants may still learn something about themselves and others, but they can be deprived of the opportunity to "own" their group's accomplishments (Blumberg & Golembiewski, 1976).

FACILITATING THE INITIAL SESSIONS

See Chapter 4 for generic tasks and strategies involved in facilitating small groups. Here we expand on those tasks and strategies most relevant to facilitating groups in which special attention is given to the human dimensions of education and health care.

Orienting learners and assessing their readiness

As in other groups, leadership tasks here include providing an overview, attending to introductions, discussing goals and expectations, and reviewing how the learners will be evaluated. Introductions can be a good time for inviting learners to talk about their lives outside of the educational program, and, as always, being diagnostic is important. Find out about the learners' prior experiences in similar groups, the extent to which they think that learners at your institution are encouraged to talk about their personal reactions to the experiences they are having, and whether they think that doing so is useful for them.

While observing the learners and being diagnostic, be aware that people from some cultural backgrounds are taught that feelings should not be shared in public; that doing so, for example, may be a sign that they are dependent on others (a negative characteristic in some cultural groups). Many men have grown up with such messages (Tannen, 1990), as have some women. You might want to explore directly the possibility that some members of your group think it's inappropriate to talk openly about feelings: "Many people have been taught not to talk about their feelings publicly. Is that true for any of you?"

Also, be aware that some members will be more able than others to verbalize their feelings, perhaps because they've had more practice doing so. For example, Tannen notes that beginning as little girls many women in our society have practice verbalizing their thoughts and feelings in private conversations with people with whom they are close. On the other hand, many boys and men are encouraged to dismiss their feelings and to keep their feelings to themselves.

Further, group members may differ in how they view seeking and giving help. Tannen (1990) suggests, "Many women not only feel comfortable seeking help, but feel honor-bound to seek it, accept it, and display gratitude in exchange. . .many men feel honor-bound to fulfill the request for help whether or not it is convenient for them to do so" (p. 65). However, many men who grow up speaking and hearing a language of status and independence resist getting help from others because it seems to put the other person in a one-up position.

None of this is to suggest that you should anticipate that men and women or people from various backgrounds in your group will act in predictable, stereotypical ways. On the contrary, we recommend that you look freshly at each person and see them all as unique. However, we do suggest that you be aware of possible factors that at least initially may make it difficult for some members to participate fully in this type of group.

Helping learners understand the purposes of reflecting on the human dimensions of becoming and being a health professional

If learners seem skeptical about the importance or appropriateness of reflecting on their personal reactions to the experiences they are having as part of their professional education, acknowledge their concerns and misgivings. Be sure they are clear about what you are inviting them to do. Consider reading a brief story or poem that illustrates the importance of self-awareness and emotional maturity in patient care and in navigating through health professions training or share your own stories. Also consider asking learners to reflect on the possible consequences in school and practice of not being self-aware and not processing painful experiences.

Creating a safe, trusting environment

Safety and trust have been recurrent themes throughout this book. Ensuring such conditions is vital when learners are revealing personal concerns and especially when they have fears about doing so. Being sure that the meeting room provides the group with privacy is a start. The following are other elements to consider.

Establish goals, roles, boundaries, and ground rules.

Learners are likely to feel more sure of themselves if they are clear about the goals and focus of the group sessions (including what topics, if any, are outside the group's concerns), what role(s) you will play (e.g., facilitator, not therapist), and what is expected of them. Consider having learners establish ground rules that will help them be as comfortable as possible. The following are some ground rules used by groups dealing with sensitive, personal issues:

- Keep confidential the identity of any patients who are discussed.
- Be courteous and respectful when others are speaking. (Don't interrupt.)
- Keep confidential anything that group members present in confidence.
- Use "I" language when offering subjective observations. (Don't presume to tell others how they are thinking or feeling.)
- Share the airtime. (Don't dominate the session.)
- Be respectful of members' requests to withhold aspects of their personal lives.

Ensure that ground rules are adhered to.   If learners break
ground rules, you can wait and see if another group member intervenes. If, however, the learner's behavior is potentially hurtful or disruptive, you might want to interrupt him without waiting for another learner to act. Often it's enough to say, "Do you remember our ground rule?"

Use an exercise to begin building trust.   An exercise or even a
carefully selected lighthearted game can help reduce tension. There are manuals and books of exercises designed specifically for groups (e.g., Pfeiffer & Jones, 1969–1989). As you select exercises or games, consider your group members' needs and levels of sophistication.

Allow time for learners to become trusting.   Typically learn-
ers are tentative when they initially come into a group when they are in Stage 1 of group formation, as discussed in Chapter 4, page 90. This tentativeness is likely to be more pronounced in groups in which learners feel vulnerable because they are being invited to talk about feelings and values. In general it's best to let learners proceed through this initial adjustment

phase at their own pace, doing what you can to foster openness and trust, without pushing too hard.

Respect learners' boundaries and limits. Effective facilitators try to be alert for group members who appear uncomfortable with a particular topic or with pursuing a topic more deeply. There is no simple formula for when to continue probing and when to ease off or stop. However, some factors to consider are the centrality of the topic to the learners' roles as health professionals, the extent to which you are willing and able to take on a more supportive role, and whether it would be more appropriate to talk privately about the matter with the learner(s) at a later time. The learners' nonverbal communications usually provide clues about the limits of what they can handle. Also, if you think the learner can be honest with you, you can say something like. "We can easily let this go, but if you want, we can explore this further, either now or later."

Support learners whose needs exceed the group's goals and resources. In a trusting environment, a student might bring up personal issues that can't be dealt with appropriately or properly in the group (e.g., because the learner's problems are so personal as to be outside the group's purposes or are so complex and serious that they require an intensive therapeutic intervention). Usually it is best to acknowledge that you have heard the learner, including any pain he or she is experiencing, but to avoid trying to manage serious personal problems in the group setting. If you are concerned that any of the group members cannot be trusted with what the learner has revealed (i.e., a member might inappropriately share the information with others outside the group), intervene as soon as possible. Let the learner who is in pain know you would like to talk further with him outside the group session. If you talk privately with the learner and determine he needs special help, try working with him to arrange for appropriate assistance.

Helping learners identify and talk about their issues

Model self-disclosure. Particularly in environments where people do not usually talk about their feelings and values, learners will likely need to see how this can be done in safe, constructive ways. Sharing one of your own experiences can be helpful, providing that doing so does not unduly shift the focus to you and your needs. For example, if the theme of the session is how members felt the first time they examined a patient, you might say (if it is true), "I was really nervous the first time I examined a patient. I was sure that he would see that my hands were shaking. What was your experience?"

Give normative permission.   Learners are likely to withhold information about themselves if they worry that their behavior may be aberrant and not well regarded. Normative permission is a strategy for letting listeners know that they are not unusual (that they are "normal"), that others engage in similar behavior or have similar feelings. ("Many students are uncomfortable posing questions about sexual behavior to patients who are their parents' age. What has your experience been?") If you make this statement in a caring, comfortable way, it also suggests that you won't be shocked or find either the learners or their responses unacceptable. You can also give normative permission by reading excerpts from health care students' and professionals' autobiographical accounts of their experiences as learners (e.g., Klass, 1987) or sensitive accounts written by others (e.g., Anderson, 1978).

Be sure to let learners know that it's not uncommon for people to feel stressed by events that they otherwise regard as positive. Also let them know that people react differently to the same event; that if they enjoyed or were relaxed during an event that their classmates found stressful, it's okay for them to talk about their more positive feelings, providing that they aren't judging their classmates' reactions but are simply reporting their own experience. (*Note*: If a learner continually reports being comfortable in situations that other group members regard as anxiety provoking, you may want to gently probe for the possibility that the learner is not being honest with herself or the group.)

Use brainstorming.   If you are leading an unstructured session in which themes are to emerge from the group but the group is having difficulty getting started, consider inviting learners to brainstorm some possible topics or issues for consideration. (Brainstorming is a process of freely expressing ideas, withholding judgments and critical reactions.) If group members still do not seem ready to identify personal issues, you can suggest that the group include issues that they think might be relevant to their classmates, if not themselves. You might also offer some topics for them to consider: "In some other groups, these were some topics that arose. . . . What do you think of them?"

Encourage learners to be as specific as possible. If other group members are to be maximally helpfully to a learner who is presenting a personal challenge or issue, and even draw personal lessons from the speaker's experience, they usually need specific details. For example, it's difficult for listeners to be fully empathic when a student is speaking in vague abstractions about being the target of a patient's anger. However, if the student paints a vivid picture of the event in language that enables listeners to actually feel as if they were there, listeners are more likely to empathize with the speaker.

Encourage learners to identify their feelings and how they dealt with them. Some learners are accustomed to routinely disregarding their feelings. So, as they talk about their experiences with patients and others, you might need to remind them to reflect on how the experience made them feel or how they are feeling now. If a learner has difficulty accessing his feelings or if you sense that he might regard his feelings as unacceptable, consider giving a personal example: "When I feel that I've been accused unfairly, I get angry." If a learner is intellectualizing, consider encouraging her to use "I" language: "I feel. . .", rather than, "It is logical to feel. . . ." Some learners manage to speak in unfeeling, intellectual ways even if they begin sentences with "I feel. . . ." If they do, help them see what they are doing, perhaps by giving them some examples. But don't push too hard. Some learners are sufficiently unaccustomed to having access to their feelings (or so uncomfortable with them) that they need several sessions before they begin to understand what you are seeking. If they are still out of reach after several sessions, that may be a signal that they might benefit from personal, professional counseling.

Show empathy. If we want learners to show empathy toward patients, we need to relate to learners empathically. Being empathic requires concentration, a willingness to suspend judgment, a capacity to tune into both spoken and unspoken communication, a sensitivity to the emotional content of messages, and an ability to see the world from another person's point of view. You can help learners express their empathy toward each other by conveying your own sense of empathy, both nonverbally (with your facial expressions) and verbally. ("That must have been very painful for you.")

Help learners be congruent in what they say and do. People who usually hide their feelings might not allow themselves to experience their feelings in the group setting. They may even try to conceal their feelings from themselves. If it appears that there is a lack of congruence between what a learner is saying and what he or she appears to be feeling, you can say something like, "You say you're angry, but I notice that you're smiling." Or, "You've described quite a frightening experience, but you seem to be making light of it." It is vital that such statements are conveyed gently and empathically, without any hint of blame or accusation. You might emphasize that being congruent is important for their dealings with patients and colleagues and deserves their time and attention.

Allow space for students to experience their feelings.   Try to allow for silences in the group. Silence can enable members to recognize feelings that might be lost if people are constantly talking. Also, silence can enable members to experience feelings that they are not yet willing or able to put into words. If learners are feeling sad and want to cry, try to make it safe for them to do so.

Include experiences that engendered positive as well as negative feelings.   Many events in becoming a health professional can engender joy. It can be especially helpful for learners to share with each other positive events that might not be as well understood by friends and family who aren't in the world of health care. However, because it's usually easier to talk about and listen to happy events, be sure not to create a climate in which learners feel pressured to share only joyful, not painful, events.

Ensuring everyone has a chance to participate

Try using a format that gives everyone an equal chance to talk. One option is to focus primarily on one or a few learners at each session, rotating the focus so that eventually everyone has a turn being the center of attention. If you will be using a more open format in which all members are invited to talk at all sessions, you may need to exert more effort ensuring that everyone participates.

As in other groups, strategies for involving all learners include asking questions, allowing time for learners to respond, and remaining neutral as you invite multiple learners to respond (see Chapter 6). Quiet members can usually be drawn out by verbally and nonverbally signaling that you want to hear from them, or you can directly ask questions of them. Initially you may choose to let some learners be quiet. However, if they continue being quiet for several sessions, you may want to speak with them privately so you can better understand their reasons for being quiet.

As in other groups, there may be members who are disruptive (e.g., interrupt others, side-talk, or seek to keep the conversation focused on themselves and their needs). If that is the case, consider the approach presented, beginning on page 94. Be more directive and forceful only as needed.

Helping learners listen to each other actively and nonjudgmentally

To be maximally helpful to each other, learners need to listen actively, both to what is said and what is unstated. They need to withhold their judgments and try seeing the world as their classmates see it. To help them achieve this level of concentration and empathy, you can model and explain this behavior, emphasizing its importance. You might also teach learners methods of quieting their minds so they can be more open to others (e.g., by briefly focusing on their own breathing or on an object in the room). Consider also engaging learners in one or more exercises in which they can practice being nonjudgmental, active listeners. For example, learners can form pairs in which Learner A spends 3 to 5 minutes telling about an event that had an emotional impact on him or her. Next Learner B tries to paraphrase what Learner A communicated, including emotional, nonverbal messages. Finally, Learner A gives Learner B feedback on the extent to which he or she felt heard and understood. Knowing that such exercises involve skills that are vital for effective patient care can increase some students' willingness to try them.

Active listening can involve tuning in to peers who are experiencing strong emotions (e.g., sadness, anger). Learners who have difficulty being in the presence of peers who are experiencing strong emotions can be helped by watching how you relate to such learners. Later, after the learner who is telling her story has finished, you might want to focus on the group members' discomfort, perhaps by saying something like, "Many people are uncomfortable when others are angry (cry, etc.) in their presence. What is it like for you?" Since students need to learn how to be available to patients who are experiencing strong emotions, consider linking the conversation to a discussion of this issue as it pertains to their work in patient care.

Helping learners support each other

When learners hear that their colleagues are having difficulty, many of them immediately want to "fix" things for them. This is particularly likely for learners in health professions programs that focus heavily on intervening and curing. The learners are typically well intentioned, but their colleague may need their support and caring, not an effort at a cure. Also, if learners rush in with ideas about how to fix the situation, they can unintentionally make it difficult for their colleague to think through and work the situation out for himself.

If you anticipate that group members are likely to have such a "fix-it" mind-set, consider having a discussion at the beginning of the first session about how colleagues can be most helpful to and supportive of each other. Invite learners to think through what can facilitate and block their talking about and then trying to deal with tough situations. Discuss how helpful it can often be just to have friends listen intently and empathically express their concern and caring. Consider pointing out that many patient problems cannot be "fixed."

Helping learners explore their possible sources of stress

Generally, people are most successful in dealing with their stress if they have some understanding of its roots. As learners talk about experiences that were stressful for them, help them reflect on why the experiences were stressful for them. In some cases, the sources of stress will be clear to them. In other cases, you might have to help them dig. For example, if a learner reports always feeling tense in the presence of a particular patient but doesn't understand why, you might invite him to consider whether this patient reminds him of a significant person in his life. If so, explore whether it's possible that he is projecting some of his feelings about this significant person onto his patient. Or if a learner isn't clear about why she gets so upset when she is asked to give maintenance care to a patient who has been in a persistent vegetative state for several years, invite her to consider whether her values are at odds with what she's being asked to do.

Helping learners identify strategies for dealing with stressful situations

After a learner has had an opportunity to talk about and process stressful situations, invite her to think through how she might approach the situation differently in the future and, if appropriate, how she might even prevent it from happening again. Encourage other learners to join you in helping their peer do this. After the learner has had an opportunity to do her own reflecting and speculating, consider inviting the other learners to offer suggestions: "Do any of you have some ideas for Helen?" Or invite the learner to consider asking her peers for suggestions: "Helen, do you want to see if any of the group members have suggestions?" Also, consider sharing your ideas and experiences.

If group members have a common issue (e.g., they think that the tight schedule for the final exams puts them under unreasonable pressure), invite them to jointly think through what they might do. If strategies for either individual or group issues lend themselves to role plays, encourage learners to rehearse what they want to do if they face the stressful event again. Also, if learners are anxious about an upcoming event, help them identify their sources of stress and some ways to eliminate unnecessary negative stress.

Some of the stressful events to which learners are exposed (e.g., the pain of a family member whose loved one is dying) are inevitable components of a clinician's life, and they must learn to deal with such events. However, there may be other sources of stress that are unnecessary or improper and need to be dealt with by the faculty. For example, hearing group members talk anxiously about upcoming exams you might realize that some exams require too much mindless memorization and are distracting from time needed for reflection and for other steps in meaningful learning. Hearing students talk about their difficulties performing certain procedures on real patients might be a clue that learners didn't have sufficient practice in simulated, preparatory settings. Hearing how students are consistently mistreated by a particular faculty member or how patients are harshly treated by some clinicians might be clues of serious abuse that must be promptly addressed by the faculty or administration (Sheehan et al., 1990).

Learners are only likely to talk about certain issues if they know that what they reveal won't be used against them. If you feel you need to discuss certain issues with colleagues or others outside of the group, you can ask the group's permission to do so in ways that protect their identities. Also, feeling strength in numbers, some learners might choose to join you in openly addressing some troubling issues.

Helping learners use the group experience for personal growth

Some people find it difficult to be fully aware of their strong feelings (particularly feelings of anger and sadness) while the experience that is engendering this emotion is occurring. Some learners are only minimally aware of even broader arrays of feelings. As we've indicated, when learners aren't in touch with their feelings, particularly strong ones, there is a risk that they will be hurtful to themselves and others, including patients.

Being helpful to patients often involves assisting them in becoming aware of their feelings and how, for example, suppressed feelings might be contributing to their health problems. To help patients become self-aware, practitioners must themselves be self-aware and able to handle their own strong emotions.

We've previously proposed some strategies for helping learners get in touch with their feelings about experiences they have had outside the group. Learners can also be helped to become more self-aware—ultimately even becoming aware of their own negative emotions as they occur—by focusing on feelings they are having within the group.

Help learners use the group as a laboratory.   If you want learners to use the group to try out new ways of functioning, talk with them about the rationale for doing so and discuss some strategies they can use. For example, suggest that during sessions learners privately practice being aware of the feelings they are experiencing. Also, encourage learners to announce if they want to practice an approach to relating that is new for them (e.g., being assertive or being quiet and reflective), and let them know that they can request the group's support in doing this.

Help learners reflect retrospectively on feelings they had in the group.   If you sense that some of the learners find it difficult experiencing their strong feelings as they happen, consider inviting them to be reflective after some time has passed, rather than during a stress-producing event in the group. For example, at the end of the session you might say, "Earlier in the session, a few group members cried when they talked about their patients who had died. How were the rest of you feeling when that happened?"

Help learners reflect on their feelings close to or during the time of the event.   If you want learners to begin reflecting on how they are feeling during stress producing events in the group, consider briefly freezing the action in the group immediately following an emotional event and inviting learners to reflect privately on what they are feeling. If you feel the group is ready, and you want them to talk about what they are feeling, perhaps start with events in the group that you suspect are engendering feelings they can discuss easily. You might ask each of them in turn to complete the sentence: "Right now, I'm feeling...." As they are more ready, challenge learners to be aware of emotions that are more difficult for them. If learners find it difficult to talk about their feelings toward others in the group, consider showing them an emotionally gripping video clip or reading an excerpt from a poignant story and then discussing how they feel. Try not to pressure learners to do things they aren't ready for. However, if learners are expected to help patients deal with strong emotions and if they don't yet seem able to do so for themselves, try finding some strategies that will help prepare them for this vital, if formidable, patient care challenge.

Help learners reflect on the possible sources of their feelings toward others in the group. As we've discussed, it's not uncommon for people to transfer to others strong feelings that they have toward significant figures in their lives. In groups, learners can project the feelings they have toward a parent onto their teacher or feelings they have toward siblings onto peers. If you suspect this is occurring and that it would be helpful for a learner to understand what is happening, consider exploring this with him during or after the group session. This is not a request for you to become a therapist or a counselor. We propose that such issues should be considered basic components of health professions education. They are appropriate and relevant for inclusion in the development of all health professionals whose work will involve helping others during highly stressful experiences.

Help learners reflect on whether difficulties they encounter outside of the group are occurring in the group. Certain kinds of relational problems are not confined to only one setting. Difficulties learners are having with patients or supervisors, for instance, might be mirrored in the group. For example, while discussing her combative relationship with a patient, a learner might realize that she has had combative interactions at times with you or others in the group. If the learner can be helped to recognize that there might be a pattern in her relationships, she may begin taking steps toward some constructive changes.

Help learners give feedback to each other.   Throughout this book we've stressed the importance of learners giving feedback to each other, and we've suggested some specific ways to help students learn to provide feedback constructively. Giving productive interpersonal feedback is particularly challenging. As Blumberg and Golembiewski (1976) observed, "It involves being in touch with oneself, as well as learning to communicate in a way that allows the other to accept what is being said. Feedback need not be acted upon by the other to be effective. Rather, feedback needs to be given in such a way that the other person can make it part of his own data bank about himself, to be used at his discretion (p. 28)." As usual one of the best ways to help members learn how to give feedback to each other in helpful ways is to model doing so yourself. They need to be reminded that providing positive feedback about what their peers do well ("Fred, I appreciate the way you make sure that everyone has a chance to talk.") is as important as providing negative feedback ("Sally, I'm bothered that you've come late to the last three sessions and have given us no explanation of what's happening.").

Helping learners summarize and reach closure

Since, as we've discussed, the group's own experience can be the focus for at least some of the session, it's important for learners to not close the session without reflecting on how they worked together, what they want to continue doing next time, and anything they want to change about the content or process, and why. You might pose specific questions. ("Is there anything we can do next time to make it easier to talk about patients and issues that are troubling you?")

As in other groups, consider having the group members summarize key things they've learned during the session. If any of them plan to take specific action before the next meeting (e.g., practice being more assertive with those in authority), having them make a public statement of these intentions can be constructively reinforcing. Make any needed plans for the next meeting. For example, if each session focuses on one or more predetermined topics, select the topics before you leave. Also, pursue the following steps.

Identify unfinished business.   Ask learners to let you know if they have any pressing issues that they need to follow up on in some way. If you are willing, let learners know that it's not uncommon for students to discover issues later, upon reflection, that they need help with (even professional help) and that they can talk with you about this after the session. You might need to assure them that seeking professional counseling can be a sign of strength and maturity and that it will certainly not reflect negatively (or even be) on their academic record (assuming that such is true, as it should be).

Discuss when and when not to be self-disclosing. It can be unsafe for learners to be self-disclosing in some circumstances. Particularly if they are relatively new to talking about personal issues and you think there is any danger that they may begin being self-disclosing outside your group in potentially awkward or hurtful situations, talk about the need for them to exercise discretion when considering being as open with others as they have been in your group.

SUMMARY

Small groups, planned and conducted appropriately, can be especially effective settings for helping learners explore and constructively deal with the many highly charged experiences they can have while becoming and being health professionals. Clinicians need to be self-aware and to reflect regularly on the feelings engendered by the work they do and the lives they lead. Without such reflection they are at risk of being insufficiently sensitive to, or even hurtful to, their patients/clients, students, residents, colleagues, themselves and their own families. Groups that include some focus on exploring the human dimensions of becoming and being a health professional can contribute to the emotional and social growth of learners, which can enhance the likelihood that they will make their way through their educational experiences successfully and emerge as effective, sensitive clinicians. Some of the key tasks involved in planning for and leading these types of small groups are summarized in the self-checklist in Appendix 10.1. For a review of the more general tasks involved in leading groups, please see Appendixes 2.1, 3.1, 4.1, and 6.1.

Appendix 10.1
Facilitating Support Groups

✔   **Did I...**

☐   orient the learners and assess their levels of readiness?

☐   help learners understand the need to reflect on the human issues
in the health professions?

>   create a safe, trusting environment?

☐   ....help learners establish goals, roles, boundries, and ground
rules, and ensure that the ground rules were adhered to?

☐   ....use an exercise to begin building trust, and allow
sufficient time for learners to become trusting?

☐   ....respect learners' boundaries and limits?

....support learners whose needs exceeded the group's goals and
resources?

>   help learners identify and talk about their issues?

☐   ....model self-disclosure and give normative permission?

☐   ....use brainstorming and encourage learners to be as specific
as possible?

☐   ....encourage learners to identify their feelings and how they
dealt with them?

☐   ....show empathy and help learners be congruent in what they
said and did?

☐   ....allow space for learners to experience their feelings?

☐   ....include experiences that engendered positive as well as negative feelings?

☐   ensure that all learners had a chance to participate?

☐   help the learners listen to each other actively and nonjudgmentally?

☐   help learners support each other and explore their possible
sources of stress?

☐   help learners identify strategies for dealing with stressful situations?

Appendix 10.1 (*continued*)

>   help learners use the group experience itself for personal growth?

☐   ...help learners use the group as a laboratory?

☐   ...help learners reflect retrospectively on feelings they had in the group?

☐   ... help learners reflect on their feelings close to or during the time of the event, and on the possible sources of their feelings toward others in the group?

☐   ... help learners reflect on whether difficulties from outside of the group affected the group?

☐   ... help learners give feedback to each other?

☐   help learners summarize and reach closure?

Epilogue

In this book we've given a good deal of attention to "process" issues and to the psychological dimensions of teaching and learning. We sought to provide some systematic ways of thinking about group facilitation and some strategies to consider when planning and conducting group sessions. In doing so, we emphasized the inevitable "messiness" of groups that are functioning effectively, how teaching is an art and so can't be reduced to simple "cookbook recipes." We emphasized the importance of being collaborative rather than authoritarian when planning and leading small groups. Giving learners responsiblity for their own and each other's learning and giving them responsibility for the group process can be unnerving to teachers who are accustomed to being in control. We hope that you were already convinced or are now convinced of the benefits to your learners of the collaborative approach.

The issues that have dominated this book typically are the concern of only a subset of the health professions teachers with whom we have worked. Indeed, we've known many health professions educators who can't imagine putting themselves in messy instructional situations, where they are not in control of events. Some of them don't even like being in situations where they might be asked questions. They can't comprehend subjecting themselves to the unpredictability inherent in the kinds of small groups we have been describing and encouraging. Also, there are numbers of our colleagues who are confused by, indifferent to, or disdainful of the human and psychological dimensions of teaching on which we've dwelled.

Yet, teaching, in our view—and as we hope you agree—just like clinical care, requires people who are highly skilled and comfortable relating to and working with people. In many educational programs faculty who are not comfortable or adept in human communications or psychological matters are still expected to teach. These teachers can usually manage to avoid attending to the human issues we've been discussing. In most programs, teachers are given sufficient control over the learning environment to shape it to their own preferences. If it suits them to do so, they can reduce or eliminate spontaneous exchanges. Yet, as we've emphasized, doing so can be damaging to learning. In avoiding messiness, such teachers are distorting the instructional environment, often at the expense of their learners. Our institutions are overdue in becoming more discriminating when selecting those who will teach and be role models for future health professional.

We must emphasize, however, that most of the thousands of health professions teachers with whom we've worked really care about teaching and their learners. They genuinely want to be helpful and most are. But many of these teachers have had little preparation for teaching and are uncertain about many of the decisions they must make. In seeking through this book to help such teachers be maximally effective, we've presented a good deal of detail. We recognize that some educators— perhaps you— may feel somewhat overwhelmed by all that we've presented. Perhaps you have a sense that there is more to being an effective small group leader than there is time, energy, or institutional support for doing. Please try to resist such a conclusion.

While presenting the many steps in preparing for and implementing small group teaching we tried to convey one dominant point and hope it is clear: the capabilities and strategies presented in this book are important but they are only part of what is needed. Equally vital is who you are. If you bring to your interactions with learners a genuine sense of caring about them and support them in their learning; if you regularly demonstrate your commitment to high-quality, humane health care; if you are a worthy role model; and if you regularly work at enhancing your effectiveness as an educator, you have the foundation on which all else depends. You are likely to make important contributions to your learners' development. Put succinctly, if you value being a teacher, are an effective professional, and treat your learners decently, you are likely to be genuinely helpful to them.

There are certainly many faculty in the health professions who are not especially given to or gifted at the human issues we've been emphasizing. We must stress, however, that there are also many teachers who are quite the opposite. They are not only psychologically sophisticated, they are so devoted to their learners and to teaching that they disregard the culture of their institutions, devoting substantial time and energy to instructional pursuits. In the absence of tangible rewards and sometimes at the expense of their career advancement, they give generously of themselves to the learners they are serving. We extend our great admiration and gratefully dedicate this book to them.

We hope we have managed to convey the sense that the many skills and understandings needed for being an effective group facilitator are learnable. If you consider taking some steps toward becoming or enhancing your effectiveness as a small group facilitator, we hope you will take seriously two messages we've encouraged you to convey to your learners: (a) meaningful learning takes considerable practice (you need to actually do whatever you are trying to learn; just reading or thinking about complex skills is insufficient); and (b) meaningful learning takes time. We hope you will be patient with yourself as you work on your facilitation skills. If you decide to modify any of your current approaches, especially any that are well-ingrained, please realize for yourself, as you must for your learners, that making such changes is neither easy nor quick.

We hope that we have helped add to your commitment to work at the lifelong task of continuously refining these skills and understandings and, most especially, that we may have helped you derive even greater joy and fulfillment from the marvelous and profound responsibility of teaching. We are confident that if you find joy and fulfillment in teaching, your students will find joy and fulfillment in learning with you.

References

Abercrombie, M. L. J. (1979). *Aims and techniques of group teaching* (4th ed.) London: Society for Research into Higher Education.

Alexander, M., Hall, M. N., & Pettice, Y. J. (1994). Cinemeducation: An innovative approach to teaching psychosocial medical care. *Family Medicine, 26,* 430–433.

Anderson, P. (1978). *Nurse.* New York: St. Martin's Press.

Argyris, C. (1982). *Reasoning, learning and action: Individual and organizational.* San Francisco: Jossey-Bass.

Ayers W. (1986). About teaching and teachers. *Harvard Education Review, 56,* 49–51.

Bales, R. F. (1950). *Interaction process analysis: A method for the study of small groups.* Cambridge, MA: Addison-Wesley.

Balint, M. (1957). *The doctor, his patient and the illness.* New York: International Universities Press.

Barrows, H. S. (1985). *How to design a problem-based learning curriculum for the preclinical years.* New York: Springer Publishing Co.

Barrows, H. S. (1986). A taxonomy of problem-based learning methods. *Medical Education, 20,* 481–486.

Barrows, H. S. (1987). *Simulated (standardized) patients and other human simulations.* Chapel Hill, NC: Health Sciences Consortium.

Barrows, H. S. (1988). *The tutorial process.* Springfield, IL: Southern Illinois University School of Medicine.

Barrows, H. S. (1994). *Practice-based learning: Problem-based learning applied to medical education.* Springfield, IL: Southern Illinois University School of Medicine.

Barrows, H. S., & Tamblyn, R. (1980). *Problem-based learning: An approach to medical education.* New York: Springer Publishing Co.

Beebe, S., & Masterson, J. (1993). *Communicating in small groups* (4th ed.). New York: HarperCollins College.

Belenky, M. B., Clinchy, B. M., Goldberger, N. R., & Tarule, J. M. (1986). *Women's ways of knowing.* New York: Basic Books.

Benne, K. D., & Sheats, P. (1948). Functional roles of group members. *Journal of Social Issues, 4,* 41–49.

Birdwhistell, R. L. (1970). *Kinesics and context.* Philadelphia: University of Pennsylvania Press.

Blanchard, K. H. (1995). Situational leadership. In R. A. Ritvo, A. H. Litwin, & L. Butler (Eds.). *Managing in the age of change* (pp. 14–33). New York: Irwin Professional Publishing.

Blumberg, A., & Golembiewski, R.T. (1976). *Learning and change in groups.* Clinton, MA: Colonial Press.

Blumberg, P., Michael, J.A., & Zeitz, H. (1990). Roles of student-generated learning issues in problem-based learning. *Teaching and Learning in Medicine, 2,* 149–154.

Bohm, D. (1993). Science, spirituality, and the present world crisis. *ReVision, 15,* 147–152.

Bormann, E.G. (1989). *Discussion and group methods: Theory and prctice.* New York: HarperCollins College.

Botelho, F.J, McDaniel, S.H., & Jones, J.E. (1990). Using a family systems approach in a Balint-style group: An innovative course for continuing medical education. *Family Medicine, 22,* 293–295.

Boud, D., & Felleti, G. (1991). (Eds.), *The challenge of problem-based learning.* New York: St. Martin's Press.

Brock, C.D. & Stock, R.D. (1990). A survey of Balint group activities in U.S. family practice residency programs. *Family Medicine, 22,* 33–37.

Brookfield, S. (1986). *Understanding and facilitating adult learning.* San Francisco: Jossey-Bass.

Brown, J.S., Collins, A., & Duguid, P. (1989). Situation cognition and the culture of learning. *Educational Research, 18,* 32–42.

Bruffee, K. A. (1993). *Collaborative learning: Higher education, interdependence, and the authority of knowledge.* Baltimore, MD: Johns Hopkins University Press.

Bruner, J. S. (1966). *Toward a theory of instruction.* New York: W. W. Norton.

Centra, J. A., & Potter, D. A. (1980). School and teacher effects: An interrelational model. *Review of Educational Research, 50,* 273-292.

Chickerella, B. C., & Lutz, W. S. (1981). Professional nuturance: Preceptorships for undergraduate nursing students. *American Journal of Nursing, 81,* 107–109.

Chickering, A. W. (1977). *Experience and learning: An introduction to experiential learning.* New Rochelle, NY: Change Magazine Press.

Christensen, C. R. (1991). Premises and practices of discussion teaching. In Christensen, C. R., Garvin, D. A., & Sweet, A. (Eds.), *Education for judgment: The artistry of discussion leadership* (pp. 15–34). Boston: Harvard Business School Press.

Christensen, C. R., Garvin, D. A., & Sweet, A. (1991). (Eds.), *Education for judgment: The artistry of discussion leadership.* Boston: Harvard Business School Press.

Coles, C. (1991). Is problem-based learning the only way? In D. Boud, & G. Feletti (Eds.), *The challenge of problem-based learning* (pp. 295–307). New York: St. Martin's Press.

Coles, J. B. (1986). (Ed.), *All American women: Lines that divide, ties that bind.* New York: Free Press.

Collins, A., Brown, J. S., & Newman, S. E. (1989). Cognitive apprenticeship: Teaching the craft of reading, writing, and mathematics. In L. B. Resnick (Ed.), *Knowing, learning, and instruction: Essays in honor of Robert Glaser* (pp. 453–494). Hillsdale, NJ: Lawrence Erlbaum Associates.

Coombs, R. H. (1978). *Mastering medicine: Professional socialization in medical schools.* New York: Free Press.

Coombs, R. H., Perell, K. & Ruckh, J. M. (1990). Primary prevention of emotional impairment among medical trainees. *Academic Medicine, 65,* 576–581.

Cross, E. (1994). (Ed.), *The promise of diversity.* New York: Irwin Professional Publishing.

Des Marchais, J. E., Bureau, M. A., Dumai, B., & Pigeon, G. L. (1992). From traditional to problem-based learning: A case report of complete curriculum reform. *Medical Education, 26,* 190–199.

DeTornyay, R., & Thompson, M. A. (1982). *Strategies for teaching nursing* (3rd ed.). New York: Wiley.

Dewey, J. (1938). *Experience and education.* New York: Collier Books.

Eble, K. E. (1988). *The craft of teaching (*2nd ed.*).* San Francisco: Jossey-Bass.

Eisner, E. W. (1985). *The educational imagination: On the design and evaluation of school programs* (2nd ed.). New York: Macmillan.

Fiedler, F. E. (1981). Leadership effectiveness. *American Behavioral Scientist, 24,* 619–632.

Fisher, B. A. (1991). *Small group decision making: Communication and the group process* (2nd ed.). New York: McGraw-Hill.

Fisher, R., & Ury, W. (1981). *Getting to yes.* Boston: Houghton Mifflin.

Fosnot, C. T. (1989). *Enquiring teachers enquiring learners: A constructivist approach for teaching.* New York: Teacher's College, Columbia University.

Foster, P. J. (1981). Clinical discussion groups: Verbal participation and outcomes. *Journal of Medical Education, 56,* 831-838.

Fox, R. D. & West, R. F. (1983). Developing medical student competence in lifelong learning: The contract learning approach. *Medical Education, 17,* 247-253.

Gage, N. L. (1984). What do we know about teaching effectiveness? *Phi Delta Kappan, 66,* 87–93.

Gibran, K. (1967). *The prophet.* New York: Alfred A. Knopf.

Goldberg, A., & Larson, C. (1975). *Group communication: Discussion processes and applications.* Englewood Cliffs, NJ: Prentice-Hall.

Hafler, J. P. (1991). Case writing: Case writers' perspective. In D. Boud & G. Felleti (Eds.), *The challenge of problem-based learning* (pp. 150–158). New York: St. Martin's Press.

Hahn, S. R., Croen, L. G., Kupfer, R., & Levin, G. (1991). A method for teaching human values in clinical clerkships through group discussion. *Teaching and Learning in Medicine, 3,* 143–150.

Hekelman, F. P., Flynn, S. P., Glover, P. B., & Galazka, S. S. (1994). Peer coaching in clinical teaching: Formative assessment of a case. *Evaluation of the Health Professions, 17,* 366–381.

Hersey, P., & Blanchard, K. H. (1969, May). Life cycle theory of leadership. *Training and Development Journal,* pp. 26–34.

Hildebrand, M., Wilson, R. C., & Dienst, E. R. (1971). *Evaluating university teaching.* Berkeley, CA: Center for Research and Development in Higher Education.

Hirsh, S. K. (1991). *Using the Myers–Briggs Type Indicator in organizations* (2nd ed.). Palo Alto, CA: Consulting Psychologists Press.

Hunter, K. M., Charon, R., & Coulehan, J. L. (1995). The study of literature in medical education. *Academic Medicine, 70,* 787-794.

Irby, D. M. (1978). Clinical teacher effectiveness in medicine. *Journal of Medical Education, 53,* 808-815.

Janis, I. L. (1972). *Victims of groupthink.* Boston: Houghton Mifflin.

Jason, H. (1962). A study of medical teaching practices. *Journal of Medical Education, 37,* 1258–1284.

Jason, H. (1964). A study of the teaching of medicine and surgery in a Canadian medical school. *Canadian Medical Association Journal, 90,* 813–819.

Jason, H. (1970). The relevance of medical education to medical practice. *Journal of the American Medical Association, 212,* 2092–2095.

Jason, H., Cohen, B. F., Friel, T., & Roland, D. (1978). *Process awareness* in the series *Teaching interpersonal skills to health professionals.* Developed for the National Library of Medicine and distributed by Centre Communications. Phone: 800-886-1166.

Jason, H., & Westberg, J. (1979.) Toward a rational grading policy. *New England Journal of Medicine, 307,* 607–610.

Jason, H., & Westberg, J. (1982). *Teachers and teaching in U.S. medical schools.* Norwalk, CT: Appleton-Century-Crofts.

Johnson, D. W. (1970). *The social psychology of education.* New York: Holt, Rinehart, and Winston.

Johnson, D. W., & Johnson, R. T. (1991). *Learning together and alone: Cooperative, competitive and individualistic learning* (3rd ed.). Englewood Cliffs, NJ: Prentice-Hall.

Johnson, D. W., Johnson, R. T., & Smith, K. A. (1991). *Cooperative learning: Increasing college faculty instructional productivity.* (ASHE-ERIC Higher Education Report No. 4.) Washington, DC: George Washington University, School of Education and Human Development.

Jones, S. E., Barnlund, D. C., & Haiman, F. S. (1980). *The dynamics of discussion: Communication in small groups* (2nd ed.). New York: Harper & Row.

Kagan, N., & Kagan, H. (1991). Interpersonal process recall. In P. W. Dowrick, (Ed.), *Practical guide to using video in the behavioral sciences* (pp. 221–230). New York: Wiley.

Kagan, N., & Krathwohl, D. R. (1967). *Studies in human interaction: Interpersonal process recall stimulated by videotape.* (Research Report No. 20.) East Lansing, MI: Michigan State University, Educational Publication Services.

Karp, D., & Yoels, W. (1987). The college classroom: Some observations on the meanings of student participation. *Sociology and Social Research, 60,* 421–439.

King, V. G., & Gerwig, N. A. (1981). *Humanizing nursing education: A confluent approach through group process.* Wakefield, MA: Nursing Resources.

Klass, P. (1987). *A not entirely benign procedure: Four years as a medical student.* New York: New American Library.

Kleehammer, K. (1990). Nursing students' perspective on anxiety producing situations in clinical settings. *Journal of Nursing Education, 29*(4), 183–187.

Knowles, M. (1978). *The adult learner: A neglected species* (2nd ed.). Houston, TX: Gulf Publishing Company.

Kolb, D. A. (1984). *Experiential learning: Experience as the source of learning and development.* Englewood Cliffs, NJ: Prentice-Hall.

Kroeger, O., & Thuesen, J. (1992). *Type talk at work.* New York: Delacorte Press.

Krysl, M. (1989). *Midwife and other poems on caring.* New York: National League for Nursing (Pub. No. 21-2286).

Lawrence, G. (1982). *People types and tiger stripes: A practical guide to learning styles* (2nd ed.). Gainesville, FL: Center for Applications of Psychological Type.

Lewin, K. (1948). *Resolving social conflicts.* New York: Harper.

Lindeman, E. C. (1926). *The meaning of adult education.* New York: New Republic.

Lowman, J. (1984). *Mastering the techniques of teaching.* San Francisco: Jossey-Bass.

Lucero, S. M, Jackson, R., & Galey, W. R. (1985). Tutorial groups in problem-based learning. In A. Kaufman (Ed.), *Implementing problem-based medical education: Lessons from successful innovations* (pp. 45–70). New York: Springer Publishing Co.

Marchard, W. R., Palmer, C. A., Gutmann, L., & Brogram, W. C. (1985). Medical student impairment: A review of the literature. *Western Virginia Medicine, 81*, 244–247.

McCormick, D., & Kahn, M. (1986). Barn raising: Collaborative group process in seminars. *Harvard Business School Publication* 8-386-025. Cited by Wilkerson, L. (1991). Becoming a problem based tutor. In D. Boud & G. Feletti (Eds.), *The challenge of problem-based learning* (pp. 159–171). New York: St. Martin's Press.

McDermott, J. F., & Anderson, A. S. (1991). Retraining faculty for the problem-based curriculum at the University of Hawaii 1989–1991. *Academic Medicine, 66*, 778–779.

McGregor, D. (1960). *The human side of enterprise.* New York: McGraw-Hill.

McGuire, C. H., Solomon, L. M., & Bashook, P. O. G. (1976). *Construction and use of written simulations.* New York: Harcourt, Brace Jovanovich.

McKegney, C. P. (1989). Medical education: A neglectful and abusive family system. *Family Medicine, 21*, 452–457.

McLuhan, M. (1967). *The medium is the message.* New York: Random House.

Moust, J. H. C., deGrave, W. S., & Gijselaaers, W. H. (1990). The tutor role: A neglected variable in the implementation of problem-based learning. In Z. M. Noomman, H. G. Schmidt, & E. S. Ezzat (Eds.), *Innovation in medical education: An evaluation of its present status* (pp. 135–151). New York: Springer Publishing Co.

Nabakov, P. (1991). (Ed.). *Native American testimony: An anthology of Indian and white relations.* New York: Crowell.

Nixon, H. L. (1979). *The small group.* Englewood Cliffs, NJ: Prentice-Hall.

Noddings, N. (1984). *Caring: A feminine approach to ethics and moral education.* Berkeley, CA: University of California Press.

Norman, G., Allery, L., Berkson, L. Bordage, G., Cohen, R., Dauphinee, D., David, W., Friedman, C., Grant, J., Lear, P., Morris, P. & van der Vleuten, C. (1989). Research in the psychology of clinical reasoning: Implications for assessment. *Proceedings of the Fourth Cambridge Conference.* Cited by Swanson, D. B., Case, S. M., & van der Vleuten, C. Strategies for student assessment. In D. Boud & G. Feletti (1991). (Eds.), *The challenge of problem-based learning* (pp. 260-273). New York: St. Martin's Press.

Norman, G. R., & Schmidt, H. G. (1992). The psychological basis of problem-based learning: A review of the evidence. *Academic Medicine, 67*, 557-565.

Osler, E. (1903). On the need of a radical reform in our methods of teaching senior students. *Medical News, 82*, 49-53.

Payne, J. (1883). Lectures on the science and art of education. Boston: Willard Small. Cited by Armstrong, E. G. (1991). A hybrid model of problem-based learning. In D. Boud & G. Feletti (Eds.), *The challenge of problem-based learning* (pp. 137-149). New York: St. Martin's Press.

Peck, S. (1987). *The different drum: Community making and peace.* New York: Touchstone.

Personnel Journal. (1974). Conscious competency - the mark of a competent instructor. July: 538-539. Cited by Whitman, N. A., & Schwenk, T. L. (1984). *Preceptors as teachers: A guide to clinical teaching.* Salt Lake City, UT: University of Utah.

Pfeiffer, W. J. & Jones, J. E. (1969–1989). *A handbook of structured experiences for human relations training* (Vol. 1–21.) San Diego, CA: University Associates, Annual Publication.

Rest, J. R., & Narváez, D. (1994). (Ed.), *Moral development in the professions: Psychology and applied ethics.* Hillsdale, NJ: Lawrence Erlbaum Associates.

Reynolds, R., & Stone, J. (1991). *On doctoring: Stories, poems, essays.* New York: Simon & Schuster.

Ritvo, R. A., Litwin, A. H., & Butler, L. (1995). (Eds.), *Managing in the age of change.* New York: Irwin Professional Publishing.

Rogers, C. (1969). *Freedom to Learn.* Columbus, OH: Charles E. Merrill.

Rogers, D. (1982, Spring). Some musings about medical education: Is it going astray. *The Pharos, 45,* 11–14.

Ross, R. (1994). Skillful discussion. In P. M. Senge, A. Kleiner, C. Roberts, R. B. Ross, & B. J. Smith (Eds.), *The fifth discipline fieldbook: Strategies and tools for building a learning organization* (pp. 385-391). New York: Currency Doubleday.

Rowe, M. B. (1986). Wait time: Slowing down may be a way of speeding up. *Journal of Teacher Education, 37,* 43–50.

Saffran, M. (1971). "Relevance" in the medical biochemistry course. *Journal of Medical Education, 46,* 1080.

Sampson, E. E., & Marthas, M. S. (1977). *Group process for the health professions.* New York: Wiley.

Scheingold, L. (1988). Balint work in England: Lessons for American family medicine. *Journal of Family Practice, 26,* 315–320.

Schön, D. A. (1983). *The reflective practitioner: How professionals think in action.* New York: Basic Books.

Schön, D. A. (1987). *Educating the reflective practitioner.* San Francisco, CA: Jossey-Bass.

Schwarz, R. M. (1994). *The skilled facilitator: Practical wisdom for developing effective groups.* Jossey-Bass.

Segal, R. (September 24, 1979). What is good college teaching and why is there so little of it? *Chronicle of Higher Education.* Cited by Whitman, N. A., & Schwenk, T. L. (1983). *A Handbook for group discussion leaders: Alternatives to lecturing medical students to death.* Salt Lake City, UT: University of Utah School of Medicine.

Senge, P. M. (1990). *The fifth discipline: The art and practice of the learning organization.* New York: Currency Doubleday.

Senge, P. M., Kleiner, A. Roberts, C., Ross, R. B., & Smith, B. J. (1994). *The fifth discipline fieldbook: Strategies and tools for building a learning organization.* New York: Currency Doubleday.

Sheehan, K. H., Sheehan, D. V., White, K., Leibowitz, A., & Baldwin, D. C. (1990). A pilot study of medical student "abuse": Student perceptions of mistreatment and misconduct in medical school. *Journal of the American Medical Association, 263,* 533–537.

Shulman, R., Wilkerson, L., & Goldman, D. A. (1992). Multiple realities: Teaching rounds in an inpatient pediatric service. *American Journal of Diseases of Children, 146,* 55–60.

Sieburg, E., & Larson, C. (1971, April). *Dimensions of interpersonal response.* Paper presented at annual conference of the International Communication Association, Phoenix, AZ, 1971. Cited by Beebe, S., & Masterson, J. (1993). *Communicating in small groups* (4th ed). New York: HarperCollins College.

Silver, M., & Wilkerson, L. (1991). Effects of tutors with subject expertise on the problem-based tutorial process. *Academic Medicine, 66,* 298–300.

Slavin, R. E., Sharan, S., Kagan, S., Hertz-Lazarowitz, R., Webb, C., & Schmuck, R. (Eds.). (1985). *Learning to cooperate, cooperating to learn.* New York: Plenum.

Strayhorn, J., Jr. (1973). Aspects of motivation in preclinical medical training: A student's viewpoint. *Journal of Medical Education, 48,* 1104–1110.

Stritter, F. T., Hain, J. D., & Grimes, D. A. (1975). Clinical teaching re-examined. *Journal of Medical Education, 50,* 876–882.

Stuart, J., & Rutherford, R. (1978). Medical student concentration during lectures. *Lancet, 8088,* 514–516.

Takaki, R. (1987). (Ed.), *From different shores: Perspectives on race and ethnicity in America.* New York: Oxford Press.

Tannen, D. (1990). *You just don't understand: Women and men in conversation.* New York: William Morrow and Company.

Tannen, D. (1994). *Talking 9 to 5: Women and men in the workplace: Language, sex and power.* New York: Avon Books.

The panel on the general professional education of the physician and college preparation for medicine. (1984). *Physicians for the twenty-first century: The GPEP report.* Washington, DC: Association of American Medical Colleges.

Thelen, H. A., & Dickerman, W. (1949). Stereotypes and the growth of groups. *Educational Leadership VI.* Cited by Jaques, D. (1992). *Learning in groups* (2nd ed.), Houston, TX: Gulf Publishing Company.

Thomas, R. E. (1992). Teaching medicine with cases: Student and teacher opinion. *Medical Education, 26,* 200–207.

Tiberius, R. G. (1989). *Small group teaching: Troubleshooting guide.* Toronto: Ontario Institute for Studies in Education.

Trautmann [Banks], J., & Pollard, C. (1982). (Eds.). *Literature and medicine: An annotated bibliography*. Pittsburgh, PA: University of Pittsburgh Press.

Tuckman, B. W. (1965). Developmental sequence in small groups. *Psychological Bulletin, 63*, 384–399.

Verner, C., & Dickinson, G. (1967). The lecture: An analysis and review of research. *Adult Education, 17*, 85–100.

Weinholtz, D. (1983). Directing medical student clinical case presentations. *Medical Education, 17*, 364–368.

Weinholtz, D., & Edwards, J. (1992). *Teaching during rounds: A handbook for attending physicians and residents*. Baltimore, MD: Johns Hopkins University Press.

Westberg, J., & Jason, H. (1991a). *Making presentations*. Boulder, CO: Centre Communications.

Westberg, J., & Jason, H. (1991b). *Providing constructive feedback*. Boulder, CO: Centre Communications.

Westberg, J., & Jason, H. (1993). *Collaborative clinical education: The foundation of effective health care*. New York: Springer Publishing Co.

Westberg, J., & Jason, H. (1994a). Teaching creatively with video. New York: Springer Publishing Co.

Westberg, J., & Jason, H. (1994b). Fostering learners' reflection and self-assessment. *Family Medicine, 26*, 278-282.

Wheelan, S. A. (1990). *Facilitating training groups: A guide to leadership and verbal intervention skills*. New York: Praeger.

Whitehead, A. N. (1916). *Address to the British Mathematical Society*. Manchester, England.

Whitman, N. (1993). A review of constructivism: Understanding and using a relatively new theory. *Family Medicine, 25*, 517–521.

Wilkerson L. (1991). Becoming a problem based tutor. In D. Boud & G. Feletti (Eds.), *The challenge of problem-based learning* (pp. 159–171). New York: St. Martin's Press.

Wilkerson, L., Hafler, J. P., & Liu, P. (1991). A case study of student-directed discussion in four problem-based tutorial groups. *Academic Medicine, 66*, (suppl. Sept): S79-S81.

Williams, P. (1995). *Workshop: Consensus decision making: The good, the bad, and the timely*. Annual Meeting of the Society of Teachers of Family Medicine.

Woods, D. R. (1994). *Problem-based learning: How to gain the most from PBL*. Distributed by The Book Store, McMaster University, Hamilton, Ontario, Canada.

Woods, D. R. (1995). *Problem-based learning: Helping your students gain the most from PBL*. Distributed by The Book Store, McMaster University, Hamilton, Ontario, Canada.

Index

Springer Publishing Company

USING THE ARTS AND HUMANITIES TO TEACH NURSING
A Creative Approach

Theresa M. Valiga, EdD, RN, and **Elizabeth R. Bruderle**, MSN, RN

This is a comprehensive sourcebook on using the humanities to teach nursing concepts. The authors, who have used the humanities to teach nursing at Villanova's College of Nursing since 1985, first give a general introduction to literature, television, film, and fine arts along with advantages and disadvantages of using each in nursing. They then describe selected nursing concepts, and provide specific examples of works of art that can be used to illustrate each. These works include a variety of art forms — novels, short stories, children's literature, poetry, films, television, music, sculpture, paintings, opera, photography, and drama. The book is designed so that nurse educators can integrate this material into standard nursing courses, and it can be used by the faculty in graduate, baccalaureate, associate degree, diploma, LPN, or staff development education.

> USING THE ARTS
> AND HUMANITIES
> TO TEACH
> NURSING
>
> A Creative Approach
>
> Theresa M. Valiga, EdD, RN
> Elizabeth R. Bruderle, MSN, RN
>
> *Springer Publishing Company*

Springer Series on The Teaching of Nursing
September 1996   256pp(est.)   0-8261-9420-6   hardcover

536 Broadway, New York, NY 10012-3955 • (212) 431-4370 • Fax (212) 941-7842

THE NURSE AS GROUP LEADER, 3rd Edition

Carolyn Chambers Clark, EdD, RN, ARNP, FAAN

This book is useful in a wide range of settings—from teaching groups to supportive or therapeutic groups to committee work with other health care providers. Simulated exercises in the book provide opportunity for practice. New to this edition are chapters on working with the elderly in groups, and on working with groups with specific problems, such as eating disorders, rape, or depression.

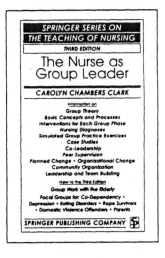

SPRINGER SERIES ON
THE TEACHING OF NURSING
THIRD EDITION

The Nurse as
Group Leader

CAROLYN CHAMBERS CLARK

Information on
Group Theory
Basic Concepts and Processes
Interventions for Each Group Phase
Nursing Diagnoses
Simulated Group Practice Exercises
Case Studies
Co-Leadership
Peer Supervision
Planned Change • Organizational Change
Community Organization
Leadership and Team Building
New to the Third Edition
Group Work with the Elderly
Focal Groups for: Co-Dependency •
Depression • Eating Disorders • Rape Survivors
• Domestic Violence Offenders • Parents

SPRINGER PUBLISHING COMPANY **SP**

Contents:

- Introduction to Group Work
- Basic Group Concepts and Process
- Working to Achieve Group Goals
- Special Group Problems
- Beginning, Guiding, and Terminating the Group
- Supervision of Group Leaders and Co-leadership
- Behavioral Approaches for Group Leaders
- Recording
- Groups for the Older Adult
- Working With Focal Groups
- When the Organization is the Group
- When the Community is the Group

Springer Series: Teaching of Nursing
1994   304pp   0-8261-2333-3   softcover

536 Broadway, New York, NY 10012-3955 • (212) 431-4370 • Fax (212) 941-7842

S *Springer Publishing Company*

INNOVATORS IN PHYSICIAN EDUCATION
The Process and Pattern of Reform in North American Medical Schools

Robert H. Ross, PhD and
Harvey V. Fineberg, MD, PhD

This book reviews continuing efforts to improve medical education in the United States and Canada. Based on a study conducted by the authors, the text and running commentaries are comprised of interviews with administrators, faculty, and students of 10 innovative medical schools. Part I compares the schools' missions, their major problems, and the faculty morale. Part II examines the schools' impetus for change and its implementation. And Part III focuses on how the innovations affect students and how students evaluate their schools' innovative curricula. This volume will be of interest to all medical educators who are concerned with the on-going debate of medical education reform.

Contents:
- Innovation Context
- School Mission
- Major Problems
- Faculty Morale
- Innovation Process
- Impetus
- Design
- Implementation
- Lessons
- Innovation Subjects
- Student Evaluations

1996   336pp   0-8261-9200-9   hardcover

536 Broadway, New York, NY 10012-3955 • (212) 431-4370 • Fax (212) 941-7842

Printed in the United Kingdom
by Lightning Source UK Ltd.
134622UK00002B/109/A